PRAISE FOR *THE BODY RESET DIET*

"I live for Harley's smoothies! They are so easy to make, help me feel full, and taste incredible!"

—KIM KARDASHIAN WEST

*"**The Body Reset Diet** makes healthy eating easier. The smoothies are simple to prepare, taste great, and are the perfect breakfast or snack when I'm on the go."*

—AMANDA SEYFRIED

*"**The Body Reset Diet** proves that you don't have to suffer, starve, or make huge lifestyle changes to lose weight, feel great, and look fantastic!"*

—HILARY DUFF

*"People think that celebrities do crazy things to lose weight, but Harley taught me that I don't have to. In **The Body Reset Diet**, he outlines simple concepts that are easy to follow even when you're working non-stop or traveling like me."*

—MARIA MENOUNOS

"I tried every diet out there and failed. Nothing was sustainable. Harley taught me how to get in the best shape of my life by eating more and working out less!"

—JORDANA BREWSTER

*"Bouncing back from having a baby isn't easy to do. But **The Body Reset Diet** helped me achieve consistent incredible results!"*

—MEGAN FOX

THE
BODY
RESET
Diet

Revised Edition

Power Your Metabolism, Blast Fat, and Shed Pounds in Just 15 Days

HARLEY PASTERNAK

RODALE.
New York

Copyright © 2013, 2021 by Harley Pasternak
Photographs © 2013 by Logan Alexander

All rights reserved.
Published in the United States by Rodale Books, an imprint of the Crown Publishing Group,
a division of Penguin Random House LLC, New York.
crownpublishing.com
rodalebooks.com

RODALE and the Plant colophon are registered trademarks of Penguin Random House LLC.

An earlier edition of this work was published by Rodale books, an imprint of Random House,
a division of Penguin Random House LLC, in 2013.

Library of Congress Cataloging-in-Publication Data
CIP data is available upon request.

ISBN 978-0-593-23216-3
eBook ISBN 978-0-593-23217-0

Printed in the United States of America

Editor: Danielle Curtis
Designer: Stephanie Huntwork
Production Editor: Serena Wang
Production Manager: Heather Williamson
Composition: Scribe, Inc.
Copy Editor: Carole Berglie
Indexer: Jay Kreider

10 9 8 7 6 5 4

Revised Edition

To my beautiful wife, Jessica, who provides me with boundless love, inspiration, laughter, and chocolate chip cookies. And my amazing kids who are even more delicious than chocolate chip cookies. And of course, to my incredible parents, who taught me to follow my passion.

Contents

Introduction   xiii

PART I
A NEW KIND OF DIET

CHAPTER **1** Why Diets Fail   3
CHAPTER **2** Why the Body Reset Diet Will Work   17
CHAPTER **3** Why Blend?   28
CHAPTER **4** Breaking Up with Sugar   38

PART II
THE FIRST 15 DAYS OF THE REST OF YOUR LIFE

CHAPTER **5** An Overview of the Body Reset Diet   53

PHASE I
CHAPTER **6** Getting Started   61
CHAPTER **7** Making the Smoothies   83

CHAPTER **8**   Learning to Move   96

PHASE II

CHAPTER **9**   Making the Transition   107

CHAPTER **10**   Easing into Resistance Training   116

PHASE III

CHAPTER **11**   Setting the Stage   135

CHAPTER **12**   Increasing the Resistance   141

PART III

THE REST OF YOUR LIFE

CHAPTER **13**   You Then and Now   157

Appendix A: Glossary of Smoothie Ingredients and Their Benefits   173

Appendix B: Smoothie Recipes   183

Appendix C: C-Snack Guidelines   213

Appendix D: S-Meal Recipes   217

Acknowledgments   285

Endnotes   287

Index   303

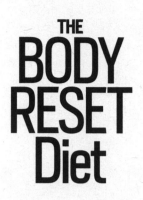

THE
BODY
RESET
Diet

Introduction

I wrote *The Body Reset Diet* in 2013 because I wanted people to see that they don't need to starve themselves or work out for hours per day to have the energy, resilience, and physique of their dreams. A person needs only common sense and a simple plan that relies on real foods and basic movements to reset one's palate, habits, and body.

I knew the plan worked, because I'd been using it with my celebrity clients, and they loved how easy it made it for them to get camera-ready. However, I was shocked to see how popular *The Body Reset Diet* became—and still is today. Since the first edition came out, it has cracked the list of top 10 diet books on Amazon numerous times and hit the *New York Times* bestseller list twice.

Why do people keep coming back to *The Body Reset Diet?* I believe it's the book's moderate approach that has continually made it stand out. After all, I wrote it to be a sane alternative to the juice-cleanse craze that had sprung up in the early 2000s. I thought of the Body Reset Diet as the anti-cleanse. The book's popularity showed that we were hungry—pardon the pun—for something more doable.

Since 2013, diet and exercise trends have become only more extreme, as we've cut out larger and larger categories of foods and have exhausted ourselves at the gym. Shortly after *The Body Reset Diet* appeared, the gluten-free craze took over, which had people running away from wheat like it was a fire-breathing dragon. Then came Paleo (no dairy, legumes, or grains), Whole 30 (same as Paleo, plus no alcohol), and keto (no carbs at all except for non-starchy vegetables), right on its heels. Now, intermittent fasting, by which you go sixteen hours a day or more without eating, or partial fasting, by which you eat only 500 calories a day one or more times a week, are the latest trends. Soon you'll be hearing about the air diet, whereby you take deep breaths only at meal times.

During this same period, extreme workouts came into vogue, and gyms specializing in high-intensity workouts sprouted across the nation. Yet our obsession with "healthy" (or what I think of as disordered) eating and go-for-broke fitness hasn't left us any better off. It's just made eating an anxiety-producing activity. With so many types of foods viewed as undesirable or even dangerous, the incidence of orthorexia nervosa—defined as an excessive preoccupation with eating healthy—has been on the rise. A 2017 study found that 49 percent of people who follow "healthy eating" accounts on Instagram have orthorexia,[1] and an earlier study from 2014 found that as many as 25 percent of college students have orthorexia.[2]

As a nation, this obsession hasn't make us any healthier, either. In 2013, 12 percent of American adults had diabetes; in 2018 (the most recent year for which data are available, as I write this), that number had risen to 13 percent. That may not sound like much of a difference, until you do the calculations and realize that it translates to an additional 3.3 million adults as so diagnosed.[3] It's even worse when you look at obesity. The percentage of American adults who were judged as obese in 2013 was 37.7; by 2018 (again, the most recent numbers available), that number was 42.4. That's an increase of 15.4 million American adults. And it makes sense. If you think the only way to get healthy is to cut out huge chunks of different types of foods and knock yourself out at the gym, you might not even try. Or, maybe you tried those radical approaches and they didn't work, so why bother with trying something new? Developing a healthier relationship with food and exercise may seem like a huge, hard task, but it doesn't have to be.

What Else Has Changed

A lot of other things have changed in the eight years since *The Body Reset Diet* first appeared, including:

Social media. While we had some social media in 2013, it wasn't then the marketing avenue for entrepreneurs it has become. Now, when you scroll through your news feed, you'll see tips from dozens of self-proclaimed health gurus, all trying to sell a supplement or a coaching program. Obtaining responsible, science-based nutrition information is hard. In the past, nutritional information wasn't widely available; now, there's too much of it, and it all comes with an agenda—to move product. We now have an enormous quantity of information and suggestions at our fingertips, but there's a lack of quality.

Before the rise in availability of social media, I could put my celebrity clients on a strict regimen so they could quickly shape up before a movie role. Now, they're posting photographs of themselves every day of the year and they require a permanent lifestyle adjustment to keep fit 365 days a year. This year-round fitness is exactly what the Body Reset Diet provides: a way to trim down quickly at the start, then tips on making your new, healthy habits a sustainable way of life forever.

The way we eat. Food delivery apps now constitute the top 40 most popular downloads in major U.S. markets, and Americans are estimated to spend $200 billion a year on takeout meals. That means people are cooking less than ever. The Body Reset Diet is a great way to get back into preparing your own meals. The recipes are quick, simple, and delicious—and you can take comfort in knowing exactly what goes into them.

My life. I've had two kids since the first edition of *The Body Reset Diet* came out, and now I'm largely focused on setting a good example for them by eating in a way that I would want them to eat. When I see people on a keto diet eating pork rinds and coconut oil, all I can think is, *Do we really think that's going to add years to our lives? Do I want my kids eating that way?*

Time is more of a premium for me now than ever before, which makes me really appreciate the ease of the smoothie. I've come to see that teaching kids how to make their own smoothies is a great way to empower them with the knowledge to provide nutritious foods for themselves for the rest of their lives. And because I had my kids later in life, I have even more reason to live as long as possible. All these factors encouraged me to take a hard look at my relationship with sugar. Not the natural sugars of fruits, but the added sugars of cookies, pastries, and candy—three food groups I ate regularly up until a couple of years ago, when I realized that I didn't want to model a sugar addiction for my kids. That led me to take a deep dive into the science of sugar and its effects on the body, and to develop a product called Sweetkick, a mint that blunts the taste of sugar on your tongue and helps you curb any sugar cravings.

Constructive feedback. While I've heard from thousands of people that the Body Reset Diet helped them lose weight and keep it off, I have also gotten some helpful suggestions that inspired me to refine the program. In particular, people reported that they got tired of smoothies after a couple of days. They craved something hot, and something savory.

Based on these developments, I've included several new features in this second edition of the book. These include:

- 12 new recipes, including 4 recipes for hot, blended soups that you can have in place of a smoothie during any phase of the diet
- Shopping lists so that you know exactly what to buy—after all, success starts at the grocery store
- More information about sugar and updated ingredient suggestions. The Body Reset Diet isn't low-carb, but it is now low-added-sugar. It also relies a little less on fruit and doesn't include any artificial sugars, which we now know are even worse than sugar in terms of contributing to sugar cravings and cueing the body to store excess weight.

I originally developed the three phases of the Body Reset Diet to give you the fastest results possible, which will motivate you to keep going. Phase I is your kick-start—it's five days of three blended meals a day; two of them are fruit-based smoothies and one is a vegetable-based soup. Phase II is the transition to more regular meals—that's when you have two smoothies and one solid meal a day. And Phase III is one smoothie and two meals. The phases haven't changed since the first edition.

However, I now realize that you don't have to start at Phase I for the plan to be successful for you. You can jump between phases depending on your lifestyle. If you need to go out to dinner, you can always start at Phase II. If you need to reset after a vacation, begin again at Phase I. Each phase caters to a different lifestyle—just pick the one that's best for you.

What hasn't changed is that the Body Reset Diet works because it helps you give your taste buds a reboot, which brings your appetite for healthy foods back into balance. It lets you experience how easy and quick it can be to make your own healthy and delicious food. The three distinct phases give you structure and a timeline. Additionally, the focus on taking a minimum of 10,000 steps a day and doing simple bodyweight exercises at home helps you develop a friendly, long-term relationship with movement. Best of all, it gives you results *fast*, so you're inspired to keep going long enough to make it a lifestyle.

You don't have to take my word for it; check out the reviews of the book on Amazon.com. Those who have reported their results rave about how they have lost 5, 10, or even 15 pounds during the first five days of the program; and over the course of the three phases, they've regained their energy and have seen some of their most troubling recurring symptoms—such headaches or debilitating PMS—improve or go away completely.

My track record is also available for anyone to see by watching *Revenge Body*, an E Network show hosted by Khloé Kardashian that helps women rededicate themselves to their own well-being; this is where I spent three seasons as one of three transformation coaches. When a contestant was assigned to work with me, we followed the Body Reset Diet. Honestly, it wasn't always an easy sell, because the contestants working with the other two trainers would be doing intense workouts, flipping tires and shaking huge ropes, right from the start; in contrast, I didn't even let my contestants into a gym for the first month. They'd say, "When are we working out?" I'd say, "Not for another month; stick to your food plan, hit your step goal, and email me at the end of the day." It seemed crazy to a lot of them, and they'd get frustrated. I'd tell them, "Just trust the process and give me five days." After three days, they'd call me and say, "I'm down six pounds!" And then I had them. Once you believe in something, it's a different ballgame. When you try this updated version of the Body Reset Diet, you'll be a believer, too.

A New Kind
of Diet

CHAPTER

1

Why Diets Fail

Many people tell me, "Harley, I've done every diet you can think of!" Take my word for it: in the long run, none of them work. Well, obviously they didn't work, or you wouldn't be reading this book. Or maybe they worked for a week or two before your weight boomeranged back to its usual number on the scale. The end result is always the same: You think you're doing everything right, and you still can't lose the weight. And after a while, you become discouraged—and why wouldn't you?

Why does nothing you've tried work? You've attempted so many diets that you can no longer open your refrigerator door without feeling a massive headache clamp down. There is SO much competing information out there, and so many contradictory recommendations, that it's no wonder we no longer have any idea what we're supposed to eat or how we're supposed to move. Eat low carb. Eat no carbs. Eat ALL carbs. Who could possibly make sense of all these competing prescriptions?

Did you know that more than half of Americans, an astonishing 52 percent, think it's easier to do their own income taxes than to figure out how to eat healthier? That's right, filing with the IRS is preferable to knowing what you should have for lunch.[1] And that's because nutritional advice these days is more confusing than the infamously complex tax code: a 2018 survey found that a whopping 80 percent of Americans say they've encountered conflicting nutrition and information.[2] (I'd say the other 20 percent just aren't looking.)

Let me tell you: It's time to stop. Enough is enough! We are listening to the wrong people telling us to do the wrong things. Who are these authorities, anyway? A lot of the TV trainers we're letting guide our fitness decisions are straight out of central casting (and I mean literally straight out of central casting), meaning they have zero credentials in the field of nutrition and have never trained anyone in their lives before their first television appearance.

There's also a tsunami of diet advice coming from the newly hatched industry of health coaching. It seems just about anyone can sign up for an eight-week online nutrition course and then hang out his or her shingle as a health coach, blanketing social media with posts and ads about a winning approach (which typically relies on products such as bars, supplements, or shakes). Now, you can't even scroll through Instagram without being inundated with conflicting nutrition advice.

People are looking to crazier diet solutions than ever before, and where is it getting them? Right back where they started—maybe even a few pounds heavier. So, before you embark on your next crazy scheme, let me explain why you keep failing and why you will see far more dramatic results from a much simpler and more sensible approach.

People often turn to the more extreme quick fixes, everything from eating like a caveman to swallowing coconut oil straight from the spoon, to spending multiple days a week eating no more than 500 calories. I mean—are you serious? Losing weight does not have to resemble an all-out death wish. The caveman lived on nuts and meat alone, but he also stayed active all day long and—oh, yeah—he generally died by age 18! In all other ways, our lives are hardly Paleolithic: we pop countless pills, eat mountains of protein bars, and obsessively log everything that passes our lips into diet apps in the hope of losing a few pounds here and there.

Weight-loss pills, many of which have been rebranded as "anti-obesity pills," are still a multibillion-dollar industry in the United States, an industry that continues to grow at 5 percent a year, despite research that has determined that no evidence exists of any single product that will result in significant weight loss.[3] Even more concerning is that some bodybuilding and weight-loss pills have been shown to cause liver damage, among other serious health issues.[4]

Whether you call them weight-loss pills or anti-obesity pills, they are so questionable that in 2020, the U.S. Food and Drug Administration (FDA) took Belviq (also known as lorcaserin) off the market because of its increased risk of causing cancer.[5] I know you want to lose weight, but it's not worth upping your chances of developing cancer. No matter what you call them, weight-loss pills just aren't worth the risk to your health.

Another sector of the market that's been exploding is meal-replacement products, including bars, shakes, and powders designed to deliver the nutrients and vitamins of a full meal in only about 200 calories and are packaged in such a way that you can grab them and go. You'll see them for sale everywhere—gyms, chiropractors' offices, online, and in grocery stores. They're taking up so much shelf space that they're crowding out actual food! The sales of these products are expected to reach *$24.5 billion* by 2025.[6] I understand the appeal: here's food that's been formulated to deliver a lot of vitamins in a shelf-stable product you can throw into your bag, keep in your desk drawer, or even eat one-handed while driving. But the very fact that these products last as long as they do means they are loaded with artificial ingredients and synthetic forms of vitamins, which taste terrible on their own. And that's why most of these bars and shakes have more sugar than a candy bar—so that you can choke them down! If they don't contain true sugar, they typically have sugar alcohols. Sugar alcohols, when taken in small amounts, don't impact your blood sugar, but if you ingest them regularly they can cause havoc in your digestive system because your body can't metabolize them properly—sorbitol, for example, is a sugar alcohol that has been shown to cause bloating and diarrhea. (No thanks! I'll take a smoothie made from whole foods any day.)

Worst of all, these meal-replacement shakes get you away from eating real, natural, whole foods, which will always be the absolute best choice for meeting your nutritional needs.

That said, there are rare times when meal replacements are helpful to keeping your nutritional intake in balance (like when you are traveling, or going through a stressful time, such as moving domiciles). I tell you how to find a decent one on page 81.

Diet and fitness apps are supposed to make it easier for us to eat healthier, but who can decide which one to use from the more than 37,000 options available in the Google Play app store?[7] Even if you do manage to find one you like, who needs another reason to reach for your phone five additional times a day? Listen, I love technology as much as the next person, but the way to better health doesn't involve hunching over your device and thumb-typing in every bite of food you eat. We need to use our bodies and brains more, not our phones!

What about cutting out an entire category of food—carbs—and gorging on fat and protein in an effort to shed weight by getting into ketosis? Have you ever smelled the breath of someone who's on a ketogenic diet? It could knock you over! (It often smells like ammonia, because all that excess protein causes your metabolism to produce ammonia as a by-product.) And reaching ketosis is only possible if you're willing to put in the time to pee on a stick, invest in a ketone-measuring device (many of which require you to prick your own finger), and pay top dollar for no-carb tortillas (that crumble when you roll them up) or locate obscure ingredients (like psyllium husks) to make your own keto buns to ensure you actually start burning fat.

When you're coping with all these issues—and I haven't even mentioned the headaches, irritability, fatigue, leg cramps, and nausea that can signify that you're starting to get into a fat-burning state—how are you supposed to carry on with the rest of your life, much less get the exercise you need to be healthy? And how can you *possibly* stay on any such extreme plan for more than a few agonizing weeks?

The answer is, you can't. That's why you're reading this book. These aggressive strategies might help you squeeze back into your favorite jeans by next Friday, but they are wreaking major havoc on your health, and the results DO NOT LAST, for a whole multitude of reasons.

Here's where the yo-yoing comes in. You lose 15 pounds by surviving (barely) on a high-fat, no-carb diet for a month, but then when you finally get exhausted and start putting real food into your poor depleted body again, your weight immediately balloons 20 pounds above your original starting point. How else is your poor confused metabolism supposed to react?

Trust me, I realize what I'm up against because I know exactly how much crazy stuff is out there. I admit that some of the better-known, more mainstream programs—with point systems and so forth—can be effective, but in many cases they take too long for the kind of results people want (and deserve), and some are also prohibitively expensive.

So, let's give up all this nutty stuff. *None of it works.* It's just crazy.

They Require Too Much Time, Effort, or Money

Many diets, including some of the healthier, moderation-based plans, fail because they ask too much of the participants' time. Whether it's attending meetings during lunch hour, writing down and adding up every bite of food consumed in the course of the day, or spending an hour of prep time per recipe five times a day, many of these diets make unreasonable demands on our already-crammed schedules. I just opened up a hot new diet cookbook, and the first recipe I saw was for a breakfast burrito—with eleven ingredients! (P.S. I made it, and it took me almost an hour. Who has that kind of time every morning?) However noble their aims, these diets simply ask too much of us. Most of us are already juggling enough responsibilities as it is.

Learning how to eat efficiently and move effectively is not rocket science, but we've complicated everything so much that it's sometimes hard to see the forest for the trees. When you don't succeed on a diet, it's not because you're a fundamentally weak person; it's because you've set yourself up to fail, with endless impossible restrictions and headache-inducing do-and-don't lists.

The other problem with most diets tends to be price. They just cost too much. Getting ready-made meals delivered to your door might be convenient, but it sure isn't cheap. The Core plan at Nutrisystem (which lets you choose your own meals instead of having them chosen for you) costs $75 a week for one person[8]—about the same as the average American spends on groceries per week for *an entire household*.[9] And some—like the Jenny Craig diet, which has an average cost of $175 per week—are even pricier still.[10] One popular partial fasting kit costs an eye-popping $249 for a five-day supply of soup, tea, and some crackers. That's $50 a day—a big financial commitment for not a lot of food, and almost no training on how to continue to eat healthy after you've finished with those (tiny) portions.

Grazing versus **Gorging**

I know that intermittent fasting has become a hot topic in the weight-loss world, but no matter how loudly its proponents crow about it, there isn't definitive science to show that it works. A 2017 randomized, controlled study (considered the gold standard of scientific research) published in the *Journal of the American Medical Association* followed obese patients over the course of a year, comparing a group of dieters who alternated between fast days (when they ate only 25 percent of their daily caloric needs) and feast days (eating 125 percent of their daily caloric needs) to a group of dieters who ate the same low number of calories every day (75 percent of their daily caloric needs) and to a group who ate normally. There was no significant difference in weight loss between the two groups of dieters; nor was there a difference in other important markers of health, including blood pressure, heart rate, or glucose or insulin levels. There were only two significant differences: the alternate-day fasters had significantly higher levels of LDL cholesterol (the bad kind of cholesterol) and were more likely to drop out of the program. So much for the life-changing magic of starving yourself every other day![11]

Another popular form of intermittent fasting is to limit the number of hours in a day by skipping breakfast, but a 2020 Chinese review analyzed the results of forty-five studies and found that skipping breakfast is associated with a higher incidence of obesity.[12] Grazing—that is, eating smaller meals more often—results in lower insulin levels, the key to any successful weight-loss plan, and the underlying principle of all my eating protocols. Several other studies support the importance of grazing over gorging to steady our metabolism and increase our body's fat-burning capacities, like one out of Spain that found teenagers who ate more than four times a day tended to have lower fat levels regardless of exercise habits.[13]

They Teach the Wrong Lessons about Food

Whether you're eating all fat, all meat, or all juice, eventually your palate will rebel against the monotony. It's perfectly natural for you to get sick of eating the exact same category of food over and over again.

The more restrictive the diet, it seems, the more likely the weight loss is temporary. According to a 2007 analysis by UCLA researchers published in *American Psychologist,* people can lose 5 to 10 percent of their weight in the first few months of a diet, but up to two-thirds of them regain even more weight than they lost within the next four or five years.[14] A 2013 review published in *Frontiers in Psychology* found that dieting is actually *predictive* of weight gain! They just don't work.[15]

Many diets ignore the fact that eating is one of the great pleasures in life. Depriving dieters of a huge range of foods makes it almost impossible for them to stay on such a limiting regimen for long. It doesn't help that most foods on these programs don't taste good. When you're living off packaged frozen entrees, or eating nothing but avocados and coconut oil all day, you're not going to look forward to your meals—and why would you? You eat this way because you want to lose weight, but after the first few days, the very idea of another frozen chicken dish and/or a bowl of guacamole eaten with cucumber "chips" makes your stomach turn, and so you stray from your plan for one meal and then another, and before the week is up you're off the program altogether.

Other diets demand we hunt down hard-to-find, exotic ingredients— say, if your local grocery store doesn't happen to carry organic free-range venison, quail eggs, or persimmons, your whole eating plan is doomed on day 1.

They Confuse Some Basic Nutritional Facts

Some diet programs focus exclusively on the old "calories in, calories out" rule, the theory being that if you expend more calories than you take in, you will lose weight, period, end of story. But diets that focus exclusively on calories and not what foods those calories are in are completely misguided. I cannot emphasize this point enough: *Not all calories are created equal.*

Fourteen hundred calories of white bread is NOT the equivalent of fourteen hundred calories of salmon. Different foods affect our bodies differently, regardless of caloric content. They make you look different and feel different, too.

A 2012 study found that following a low-fat diet can slow down your metabolism, which makes weight loss more difficult.[16] A 2019 review found that a higher-protein diet was significantly better for keeping weight off in the long term than either a high-fiber or low-glycemic diets.[17] So, losing weight is not a simple matter of caloric arithmetic; nor is it as easy as cutting out entirely or focusing exclusively on one type of food. You also have to consider WHAT you're eating, not just how much of it.

Far too often, diets deprive us not only of calories but also of the foods we need in order to live at the top of our game. If, for example, you're on a juice fast, you're not getting ANY protein, healthy fats, or fiber—and your body needs all these nutrients to function. Because you're depriving your body, you'll probably be hungry, miserable—and extremely vulnerable to falling off the wagon. We also don't take in enough liquids, and many of us live in a state of semi-dehydration, which our bodies far too often confuse for hunger, which causes us to eat more.

They Push Exercise Too Much

Never thought you'd hear that from a fitness professional, did you? Overexercising can be a real problem. First off, no amount of exercise can undo the effects of a bad diet. Do you know how many minutes you have to do on an elliptical trainer to offset the caloric burden of a single slice of cheesecake? Up to an hour and a half. As Gary Taubes put it in his well-argued book *Why We Get Fat*, "very little evidence exists to support the belief that the number of calories we expend"—that is, how much we work out—"has any effect on how fat we are."[18]

I believe it's because our over-the-top workout habits end up super-charging our appetites, ultimately causing us to consume even more calories than we would have if we'd stayed home and skipped the gym. Taubes once again states the case plainly: "Increase the energy you expend and the evidence is very good that you will increase the calories you consume to compensate."[19] Put in the simplest terms possible, the harder you work out, the hungrier you'll be and the more you will eat. But if you want to lose weight, increasing the number of calories you're taking in is counterproductive, at best.

I started thinking about this seeming contradiction more and more in the summer of 2009, when *Time* published a cover story called "Why Exercise Won't Make You Thin."[20] The gist was—hey, it's great that you go to the gym, but if you leave the gym famished and hit the all-you-can-eat buffet on your way home, you're still going to gain weight, simple as that.

So, if exercise isn't the key to weight loss, why have so many popular fitness programs failed to get this message? Turn on your TV and look at all the current exercise infomercials out there; ever tried working out with that drill sergeant shouting orders at you to do nearly impossible types of exercise at nearly impossible levels of intensity with no regard for the possibility of injury? Many of these programs are way too difficult, way too intense, and there's just no method to the madness. I myself am in great shape and can't do most of these exercises! Why is there a program based on chin-ups when only a fraction of the population can actually do these incredibly advanced exercises?

Far too often, this radical approach to exercise—the extreme boot camps, the triathlon training, the high-intensity fitness classes that emphasize the number of reps completed in a certain amount of time over proper technique—has another unfortunate unintended consequence. It can lead to an explosion in sports injuries, back problems, and tendinitis, which in turn impedes one's ability to maintain physical activity over the long term. Our ever-growing passion for marathons, triathlons, ultramarathons, and other "extreme endurance exercise" can have serious negative effects on our bodies, leading to scarring of the heart tissue, particularly in men, that can contribute to heart failure, as a 2017 study found.[21] Our love of intense workouts—from spinning to CrossFit—has resulted in a spike of a potentially life-threatening condition called rhabdomyolysis, or rhabdo for short, where muscle cells explode and leak their contents into the bloodstream, an event that then taxes the kidneys and leads to extreme muscle pain and weakness, as well as brown urine. The rise in incidences of rhabdo caused one medical doctor to call it a "public health concern" in a 2016 article in the *American Journal of Medicine*.[22] We are pushing ourselves too far, and for no good reason.

They Don't Make Us Exercise *Enough*

The flip side of the tendency to overexercise is that most of us don't exercise *enough*—even those of us who devotedly attend a kick-ass spin class after work every night. Sound like a contradiction? It's not. Regular gym attendance can in no way compensate for an otherwise completely sedentary lifestyle. And for far too many of us, sedentary is the norm. Thanks to the internet, cellphones, and all the other technologies that rule our days, most of us can get through the workday without once getting up from our desk. We can buy our clothes and even our groceries without taking a step. These technological advances have made our workdays more efficient, but what are they doing to our bodies?

If we drive everywhere and sit at a desk all day, then return home to sit on a couch all night, we are going to gain weight. Period. It really is that simple. A landmark 2012 Finnish study found that, while regular exercise is important for health, long bouts of physical inactivity can be hazardous *even if the person also exercises.*[23] Additionally, a 2019 study by researchers at the Cleveland Clinic analyzed the health records of approximately 122,000 patients who had undergone treadmill testing at the clinic from 1991 to 2004. They found that those who were the most unfit had a higher risk of dying than people who smoked, had hypertension, or had diabetes—a LOT higher: the least fit had a risk of dying that was four times higher than those who exercised regularly.[24] The message is clear: get moving, or die early.

Despite this clear correlation between an active lifestyle and health, most diet plans fail to take into account the importance of regular movement in maintaining a healthy weight. When you are starving yourself half to death, you seldom have the energy to move, and when you fail to move, you quickly lose your lean muscle tissue, which in turn makes your resting metabolism go down, which in turn makes it harder for your body to lose weight. Seriously, try doing any sustained exercise—much less doing daily household chores—when you haven't properly fed your body in almost two weeks. It's not going to happen.

Again, the internet and our culture of consumption are not helping the cause much. Far too many of us fall into the trap of purchasing ridiculous fitness products advertised on TV or on social media—you know, like that electrical stimulating belly belt, or ridiculous devices like the Shake Weight or Spin Gym. I'm sorry, but the only calories you'll burn with these rip-offs will happen when you get your credit card statement and your heart rate soars because you realize you spent actual money on this junk!

The Number on the Scale Doesn't Move Fast Enough

This is a big one, and the hardest for me in particular to acknowledge. I fought the good fight for a long time, saying over and over that it's far better to lose half a pound a week over twenty weeks than to drop 10 pounds in a week. When I moved to Los Angeles almost twenty years ago, I started to see just how desperate people were to lose weight *right away,* in the snap of a finger. When my voice of reason and logic failed to penetrate their sense of urgency, I would lose these clients, who would go off to try the latest overnight body-transformation scheme. I saw even more of this desperation when I began to work with women on the *The Revolution* and *Revenge Body with Khloé Kardashian*—and, as I've said, I saw the positive side of this mindset as well, which is to say that the ones who lost the most weight right away were the ones most likely to stick with the program, even after those shows were over.

I've since accepted that people get psychologically frustrated when their progress is too slow. You are enduring what feels like Herculean sacrifices to improve your body, but that number on the scale just refuses to budge. So, yes, you will inevitably feel discouraged, and you have every right to be frustrated—not only at your body but also at this stupid diet that's making you suffer for no reason. What's the point of depriving yourself of all the foods you love if you have nothing to show for it?

The answer is: THERE IS NO POINT. You *can* get the body you want and deserve without going to hell and back. I'll show you how.

2

Why the Body Reset Diet Will Work

So, is there really a diet out there that's actually *good* for our bodies? That works with—instead of against—our bodies' metabolism, that keeps our appetites satiated and our taste buds entertained, that accommodates our insanely overstuffed schedules while also yielding amazingly fast yet sustainable results? Is there a way to lose weight quickly without risking a trip to the emergency room or guaranteeing that you'll balloon up to an even larger size when it's all over?

Yes, yes, and yes. I've created the Body Reset Diet precisely to help you where all those other diets have let you down. Trust me, you do NOT have to sacrifice your health or put your life on hold, or empty your bank account to finally get the body you've always wanted. You can eat delicious foods, exercise only a few minutes a day, have a huge amount of energy, and feel better than you ever have before, all the while shedding pound, after pound, after pound.

My plan is completely different from anything you've ever tried before—and *way* more effective. It will help you lose weight right away, and keep that weight off in the years to come. So, just stick with me for the next 15 days and I promise that when it's all over your friends won't recognize you. You might not even recognize yourself!

Whatever brought you to pick up this book, *The Body Reset Diet* is going to revolutionize the way you think about dieting—and revolutionize your body in the process. You'll:

- Lose fat quickly and safely
- Experience a massive energy boost
- Enjoy improved overall health
- Feel as amazing as you look

Yes, I'll say it again: By the time these 15 days are up, you will look and feel *dramatically* better. And to get there, you won't have to suffer even for a second. You will quickly learn that losing weight is not a form of punishment.

You will also be finding that happy medium on the exercise front: an element of healthy living that most diets either ignore completely or dangerously overemphasize. On the Body Reset Diet, you will learn the importance of moving consistently throughout your day for optimum health. It's MUCH more important to move regularly than to throw yourself into some radical exercise regimen that will probably land you in the orthopedist's office before the year is up.

Unlike other diet plans, you will be taking care of your body every step of the way. The secret to the Body Reset Diet is that it kick-starts rapid weight loss *without* depleting you of vital nutrients or quality of life. From the very beginning, you'll be getting all the nutrients your body needs to thrive.

There will be no attempts at starving yourself thin here—repeated studies have shown that such efforts inevitably backfire, anyway. Five times a day, you'll be filling yourself with foods that are as satisfying as they are delicious. Even in the first five days, you'll never feel hungry because you'll be eating such a high volume of food at regular intervals throughout the day. The food you'll be eating will also be extremely nutrient dense, and your body will be using every calorie you take in.

On the Body Reset Diet, you can expect to see rapid weight and inches lost within the first five days, and this is as much a result of a boosted metabolism as of calorie reduction. Other diets, in contrast, deprive users of various nutrients at the expense of their metabolism. The key to avoiding the seesaw ups and downs of most diets is to never put your body into this self-defeating deprivation mode.

It's critical to understand that we don't lose weight by denying ourselves food; on the contrary, we lose weight by eating small meals around the clock. Whatever you've been taught, the easiest way to take off the pounds is to eat *more* often, not less. After all, it's when we get really, really hungry that our insulin dips and spikes, which causes our bodies to store food as fat. That's also when we lose sight of our best intentions—and lose control. We end up eating more food than we intended, and certainly more than we needed.

To make your metabolism more efficient, you need to get into the habit of grazing instead of gorging. Eating five times each day on the Body Reset Diet shifts your metabolism into high gear, meaning you'll burn even more calories and shed more fat 24/7—yes, even while you're fast asleep!—without throwing your body into confusion.

The Body Reset Diet will teach you how to maintain consistent blood sugar levels and never experience those dangerous dips in energy that lead to bingeing and general exhaustion and despair. Eating regularly helps tame your appetite and control cravings, and the high amounts of fruits and veggies you'll be consuming will overload you with bio-available nutrients that unlock your metabolism's true potential.

Perhaps the biggest difference between the Body Reset Diet and the rest of those trendy diets is that my plan is designed for the long haul, to provide guideposts not just for the first 15 days but also for the rest of your life.

Why Diets Fail	Body Reset Diet Solution
The number on the scale doesn't move fast enough.	In the first phase of the Body Reset Diet, you can expect to see rapid weight loss. You'll feel satiated throughout the day and motivated to stick with the plan.
They encourage the false assumption that all calories are created equal.	The Body Reset Diet explains what foods are to be consumed and WHY. By understanding the importance of a high-protein and high-fiber diet, you're empowered to make smarter eating decisions moving forward.
They take up WAY too much time.	It doesn't get easier than throwing raw or frozen ingredients into a blender. It's faster (and much cheaper) than calling for delivery or going out to eat in a restaurant.
The extreme calorie restriction they recommend leads to a state of semi-starvation.	On the Body Reset Diet, you'll consume 3 daily meals and 2 daily snacks made up of protein and fiber that will provide adequate calories and all the nutrients you need to thrive.

Why Diets Fail	Body Reset Diet Solution
They require too many changes at once.	The Body Reset Diet is easy to use and easy to implement, and the changes are incorporated gradually.
They lead to food exhaustion and boredom with a limited range of ingredients, or they require exotic, hard-to-find ingredients.	The Body Reset Diet provides a multitude of delicious, filling recipes that are fun to prepare and consume, and it's built around foods you can buy at any supermarket.
They cost too much.	Once you start blending, you will start saving big money on this diet by using seasonal and/or frozen foods. You'll also save by not eating out in restaurants as much.
They don't set a good example for your kids.	Instead of teaching them to fear entire categories of foods, the Body Reset Diet helps you model a balanced, whole-foods–based diet. Making smoothies with your kids is also a great way to empower them to make their own healthy breakfasts and snacks and train their taste buds to appreciate the taste of real food.
It's impossible to live your normal life on them.	How can you go out to dinner if you're not eating that day? How do you attend your kid's pizza party if you're not eating carbs? The S-meals in the Body Reset Diet are all things you can easily find a facsimile of on most restaurant menus, and if your life requires you to go out to dinner regularly, you can always start with Phase II so that you can eat out. Also, with two "free" meals a week once you're in maintenance mode, you won't have to bring your own celery sticks to any celebratory meals ever again.

Are you ready to get started on the easiest, most rewarding diet you've ever been on?

Why You Can Trust
That the Body Reset Diet
Will Work for You

I have ten years of undergraduate and graduate education in nutritional science and exercise physiology; I spent years consulting for the military on the impact of food and drugs (like caffeine) on human performance; and twenty years in my practice as a fitness trainer (a field in which I am certified by the American College of Sports Medicine and the Canadian Society of Exercise Physiology, and hold the title of IDEA Master Trainer). I've also written seven bestselling books about diet and fitness. It's a lot more than I can say about most of the high-profile "experts" who are dictating the health decisions too many people are making today.

But even with all my experience, I had more to learn. As I've mentioned, in 2013, I had the privilege of hosting an ABC daytime talk show called *The Revolution,* and in 2017, I began my stint on *Revenge Body with Khloé Kardashian.* Being on these shows were two of the most rewarding experiences of my professional career. The amazing women I met helped me rethink my whole weight-loss philosophy.

I had always worked with entertainers and actors, a demographic that certainly has its unique challenges. But it wasn't until I was on these shows that I was able to work with—and get feedback from—the average American. It made me think about the accessibility and price of ingredients, and how many people are either cooking for one or also cooking for their families and don't want to have to cook two meals every night while on their quest for better health. The folks I worked with on these shows all had different emotional and physical histories, too, and I saw how much psychology and a history of weight struggles have to do with success in the realms of diet and fitness. It made me simplify my process, and focus on creating stages so that, no matter where you're starting from, you can see results quickly, which will help fuel your desire to keep going.

It's my education, and the wide range of people whose bodies and minds I've helped transform over the past twenty years, from Halle Berry and Jessica Simpson to single-mom schoolteachers, that has led me to understand the seriousness of the crisis we're facing. Let me tell you, I know exactly what you're going through—whether you need to lose a ton of weight or just those last stubborn 5 pounds—and you have no idea where to begin. That's what I'm here for. Stick with me for the next 15 days and you will see amazing, dramatic results in your energy level, in your health, and most noticeably in your body. To get there, first we have to wipe the slate clean. Rethink everything you've ever been told about how to lose weight. Press Reset. Start over.

What You Can Expect to Do on the Body Reset Diet

The Body Reset Diet lasts just 15 days, broken into three distinct 5-day phases. By the end of the 15 days, you may be shocked by how much your body—and your whole perspective on diet and exercise—has changed. You'll:

- Spend less time and money than ever before on food
- Eat more fruits and vegetables than ever before—without even noticing (and trust me, this is coming from someone who *hates* vegetables)
- Prime your metabolism to work with you around the clock

- Give your body access to more fat-burning, usable nutrients than ever before

- Burn fat nonstop, all day long (and even while you sleep), without ever setting foot in a gym

- Sculpt your body in just a few minutes a day, with no equipment necessary

What You Can Expect to Learn on the Body Reset Diet

This plan isn't just limited to the next 15 days. A big part of it is about educating you about health and fitness so you'll know why you're eating and moving in this way. The more you understand today, the better you can live tomorrow. I want you to take away more than just a hot body from this book! You'll learn:

How to make the right nutritional decisions. I want you to learn not only *what* is in your meals but also *why* you are eating those particular ingredients in those particular combinations. Why is it so important to eat fiber at every meal? Why is a meal not a meal without protein and fiber? Why are people who regularly eat fruits and vegetables so much thinner than those who don't? Understanding the difference between good and bad fats, and simple and complex carbohydrates, will empower you to make the right nutritional decisions for the rest of your life.

How to create structure within your day. Instead of eating on the go or grabbing lunch from a vending machine whenever you feel that first stab of hunger (or whenever you feel bored or distracted), you'll learn to schedule the times you eat in advance and to make a ritual out of your meals that allows you to actually enjoy them. And guess what? By planning your meals ahead of time, you'll also save both time and money. You'll be less likely to run out of crucial ingredients, and less likely to order over-priced, greasy takeout at the last minute because you can't think of anything to make that night. Because you'll enter the store armed with a list, you'll be less tempted to fill your cart with unhealthy, impulse-item ingredients.

How to become a more efficient eater. Make your calories count. Build your diet around nutrient-dense high-volume foods so that your body will adapt to getting more out of less. A blender is one of the best ways to maximize the bioavailability of foods, which is one reason it's the centerpiece of the Body Reset Diet. It also happens to be one of the easiest ways to prepare food.

Perhaps most of all, I want you to get it in your head that YOU DO NOT HAVE TO SUFFER TO LOSE WEIGHT!

Like I said, forget everything you've been told. Weight loss should not be a form of punishment. It is your *reward* for working hard and making the right decisions. It's a real tragedy that in our all-out, apocalyptic struggle to shed the pounds, we've come to regard food as our enemy. Forget that! Food is one of the great pleasures in life, and you *can* eat well and still lose weight; in fact, eating well is the only way *to* lose weight. So, let's forget everything we know about nasty "diet food" and bring the joy back into eating again.

Life is difficult enough already. Your diet should be easy—and fun.

"By the time I worked with Harley on *Revenge Body*, I had been sober for more than 10 years. Prior to that I had spent most of my life addicted to drugs. After years of drug abuse, my metabolism was basically nonexistent and it was very difficult for me to keep weight off. About a year before I met Harley, I developed a crippling anxiety disorder. While the medication I took to manage it did make me feel better mentally, it also caused me to gain 50 pounds. I also didn't have a whole lot of healthy habits as far as diet and exercise went.

"Harley wasn't daunted by my challenges. He even used to joke how he loved working with folks in recovery because our natural inclination toward addictive behavior means we can get just as addicted to exercise and a healthy lifestyle as we could to any substance. Although I was inspired by the way he looked at things, Harley and I did not get along in the beginning. It's actually funny to think back on it now because we ended up becoming great friends, but in the beginning we butted heads so frequently that I am SURE I annoyed the hell out of him. But still, he persisted.

"I couldn't understand how drinking smoothies full of fruit and just walking around was going to be beneficial. It just didn't make sense to me. I was also so overweight and so out of shape that doing the 10,000 steps a day seven days a week was incredibly painful. I got shin splints, pulled muscles, and worst of all I developed plantar fasciitis, which brought with it a level of pain I can't even put into words. It was hard and it was painful and I hated every minute of it, but Harley has no tolerance for BS! He gifted me a pair of running shoes and told me where to get the proper inserts to support my plantar fasciitis and was not excepting any excuses. And so, I did as I was told.

"It took a little while to see results start but then it all started coming together really fast. As the weight came off I had less pain. I was completing my steps sooner, and was able to walk even more than 10,000 steps. I felt better and better every week. I was losing weight, I was losing inches, I was becoming more comfortable in my body, I was becoming more confident in myself, and the more all that happened the more driven I felt. By the time my 10 weeks with Harley were over I had lost 36 inches all over my body and 42 pounds total.

"At the beginning of our time together I was a little thrown off by the fact that Harley takes a very hands-off approach with his clients. But over time I realized that he was setting me up to be self-sufficient, to achieve and maintain results without him needing to guide me every step of the way. He was teaching me how to take care of myself for life. About two years after I worked with Harley I decided to get off my anxiety medication. I ended up gaining 40 pounds. I immediately started Harley's program over again from the beginning, but this time, I could do more exercises right from the start—even though I had gained weight, my strength and my stamina were still intact. Within six months of starting over, I lost 52 pounds. I actually weigh less and am healthier today than I was when we wrapped the show.

"Harley taught me a way of taking care of myself and my health and my body that is realistic and sustainable and I am forever grateful to him."

—JESSY, *REVENGE BODY* CONTESTANT WHO LOST 52 POUNDS
AND LEARNED A LIFETIME OF HEALTHY HABITS

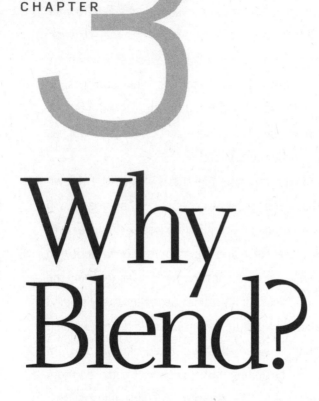

3

Why Blend?

Before we get into the nitty-gritty of the three phases, let's talk about the main tool you need to get started: a blender. Most of us have one already, but what do we use it for? Maybe a milkshake every month or so, or perhaps some frozen margaritas when it's hot out.

Well, guess what? This underappreciated kitchen gadget will be an indispensable part of getting you back on the road to wellness. Learn to love your blender and your body will thank you for it. Blending is one of the quickest, most convenient ways to prepare food. Anyone can do it, on any schedule. You won't have to deal with setting timers or waiting for water to boil; there will be no julienning or defrosting. With a blender, you just throw everything into the jar and press Start. Using my guide–

lines for a complete smoothie, you can create an entire meal in under 90 seconds.

A blender gives you access to a wide range of good-for-you ingredients, putting all sorts of healthy foods at your fingertips. Blending makes the intimidating easy: with the help of a good blender, it's zero effort to get more fruits and vegetables into your diet than you ever thought you could. Blenders are also good tools for disguising what might not be your all-time favorite flavors. For example, you might not like how spinach tastes on its own (I know I'm not the biggest fan), but how about when it's blended with some mangoes or blueberries? You won't even be able to recognize the leafy green superfood; it's the fruit flavors that dominate.

Forever Young:
Fruits and Vegetables

Eating a lot of fruits and vegetables benefits your whole body. Vitamin A, found in carrots, cantaloupe, and lettuce, is known to boost immune system function. The mind–gut connection is also something to consider: a 2018 study found that young adults who ate more raw fruits and vegetables than processed fruits and vegetables (think applesauce and fruit juice) had fewer symptoms of depression, a more positive mood, and higher life satisfaction.[1] And yes, fruits and veggies also promote your eternal youth and beauty: women who eat a lot of vitamin C–packed foods like oranges and guava have fewer wrinkles than women who don't, according to a study published in the *American Journal of Clinical Nutrition* that tracked the diets of more than 4,000 American women ages 40 to 74.[2] Another study assessed the diets of 3,775 Norwegian young adults, and suggested that raw veggies might reduce breakouts by as much as 30 percent.[3]

Best of all, your body can actually use these ingredients when they're in blended form, because blenders break down food into molecules that are efficiently metabolized and readily *bioavailable*—that is, absorbed into your body in a manner it can use. And while this may not be the most appetizing example, a study done with chicken livers measured how blending time impacted the bioavailability of nutrients, particularly iron. The study found that particles processed in a blender for 6 minutes resulted in more than twice the iron of chicken liver blended for just 60 seconds.[4]

Blending is especially helpful for some vegetables—like broccoli—that are really fibrous and thus harder to break down. Running your broccoli through a blender means it is essentially predigested (since chewing is part of the digestive process) and therefore easier for your body to break down and assimilate its nutrients. Blending vegetables also helps you eat a greater quantity of them—think about a basketball-sized mass of spinach: once it's cooked and then blended, it could fit into the palm of your hand. That means the nutritional density of your finished soup is very high.

Blending versus Juicing

So, you're asking, if blending is so great, isn't juicing better? Juicing takes more time and costs more money, so surely it's healthier—right?

Wrong, wrong, and wrong again. Contrary to conventional wisdom, juicing is *far* inferior to blending, and not just because blenders are infinitely easier to operate and clean than juicers, which also happen to be a headache to assemble and disassemble (and who can possibly keep track of all those parts?).

Juicing also requires a great deal more produce to achieve the same

Choosing the Right **Blender**

Though the first commercial blender wasn't introduced to the market until the 1930s, the concept of a blended beverage is millennia old—just look at the Indian lassi, a drink of blended fruit and yogurt. These days, blenders are as high-tech as it gets. You can pulverize just about anything in your kitchen, from whole nuts and sesame seeds to full apples and carrots. There are no limits.

When choosing the right blender, here are a few things to consider:

- A minimum of 500 watts, to make sure you have enough power to blend harder produce or nuts. Ideally, you will want even higher power than that.

- A large jar (the blender container) that's dishwasher safe, to accommodate smoothies prepared as meal replacements (produce like spinach takes a lot of space).

- A heavy base for stability.

- A design that's easy to clean (such as a unit with a flat control panel versus multiple buttons that's hard to wipe around).

- Capability to grind seeds or cacao beans, and so on (coffee grinders can do this, but you benefit if your blender already can do this).

- On top of these, while it's not a "must-have," if your blender can also crush ice into a nice "shaved ice" consistency, you can do a lot more with your blender—such as delicious fruit or green cocktails!

Depending on your budget, you can invest in an expensive blender (like Vitamix or Blendtec) or choose from some great budget blenders.

My smoothie recipes can be easily modified for all types of blenders. And no matter which you pick, a good blender is a good long-term investment in your health.

quantity of liquid as an equivalent blended beverage—sometimes three to five times as much. That's because only a small portion of the fruit goes into the finished product of the juice. Have you ever seen how much they throw away at juice bars? They discard all the fibrous parts of the fruit or vegetable that hold all the nutrients.

With blended smoothies, all of those nutrients, and the entirety of the fruit or vegetable—including the all-important fiber—are going straight into your body. The waste associated with juicing isn't just a concern from a financial or environmental perspective. It's not doing your body any favors, either. Far from being bad for you, the fibrous parts excluded from juices are actually the most nutritious components of the plants! As my old professor Dr. Glynn Leyshon at the University of Western Ontario once quipped, "Since most of the nutrients and nearly all of the fiber is in the skin, seeds, and pulp," he said, "you're better off throwing out the juice part and drinking the rest!"

That's right. Once all the fiber has been removed, most juices are left with large and extremely unhealthy quantities of sugar. Some juices have an even higher sugar content—and in many cases more calories— than sugary sodas, and that's saying something. Just think: making a cup of orange juice takes the juice of, say, three oranges, and drinking it is much less filling and *way* less nutritious than eating a single orange whole. If you don't believe me, try comparing the nutrient profile of a cup of orange juice (132 calories, 31 grams of carbohydrates, 0.4 gram of fiber, 25 milligrams of calcium, and 64 milligrams of vitamin C) with that of a cup of solid orange segments (82 calories, 19 grams of carbohydrates, 4.5 grams of fiber, 82 milligrams of calcium, and 102 milligrams of vitamin C).

Apple Juice versus Blended Apple Beverage

It's not just oranges where the actual fruit is healthier than the juice. Let's take a look at the difference between sticking an apple in the blender and drinking it (what I'm calling a "blended apple beverage") versus a cup of apple juice from a bottle.

	"Pure" Apple Juice (16 fl oz)	Blended Apple Beverage (16 fl oz)
Calories	240	120
Fat	0 g	0 g
Protein	0 g	0.75 g
Sugar	57 g	19 g
Fiber	0 g	3 g
Cost (approximate)	$2.75	$0.65

Far and away, the healthier option of the two—the drink that's lower in sugar, lower in calories, higher in protein, and higher in fiber—is the blended apple. All its nutrients remain intact, and because you're not throwing anything away, the blended apple is also the cheaper option, coming in at only about 32¢ per 8-ounce cup. Research has even found that consuming fruit that has been blended by a high-speed blender (the style I recommend) actually has significantly *less* of an impact on blood sugar than eating an equivalent amount of that same fruit in whole form![5]

The Fiber Factor

Let's look a little more closely at the reasons you should always reach for a blended apple over a juiced one. The most important one bears repeating: blended drinks, unlike juiced ones, contain both the juice and the pulp from your produce, and the pulp contains the number one nutritional benefit of the drink, fiber.

In its natural form, almost every fruit and vegetable has some fiber content, but we don't eat nearly enough produce, and our diets are frighteningly deficient in fiber. The American Dietetic Association recommends women consume a minimum of 25 grams of fiber a day and men consume at least 30 grams, but most Americans get only about 10 grams a day—roughly one-third of the recommendations. Ideally, I'd like you to get at least 40 grams of fiber in your daily diet.

More fiber leads to more weight loss—it's just that simple. The vast majority of studies have concluded that more dietary fiber yields greater

Liquid **Energy**

Various studies indicate that liquid meals can be more filling than solid meals. The Body Reset Diet capitalizes on this science to produce impressive weight-loss results with a combination of smoothies and a high intake of other liquids. One study shows that when participants ate a first course of soup before a lunch entrée, they reduced their total calorie intake at lunch (soup + entrée) by an amazing 20 percent, compared to when they did not eat soup.[6] That's one reason you'll be drinking so much water in addition to your smoothies—because a high volume of liquids helps keep your body detoxified and your stomach full.

More **Fiber Facts**

Fiber extends your life span. When the National Cancer Institute and the American Association of Retired Persons (AARP) studied dietary fiber intake in relation to total mortality, as well as death from specific causes, they found that both men and women with the highest fiber intake—specifically fiber from whole grains—had a significantly lower risk of death.[7]

Fiber fights disease. A 2010 study found that diets rich in soluble fiber can help reduce the inflammation that can lead to obesity-related diseases like diabetes and heart disease. The same study found that fiber can help strengthen the immune system.[8]

Fiber keeps your pipes clean. Fiber is perhaps the most important nutrient for maintaining proper bowel health. It bulks up your diet and helps avoid constipation and all the unpleasantness that entails.

satiety and lower incidences of hunger. In fact, adding 14 grams of fiber a day has been shown to lead to a 10 percent decrease in caloric intake and an increased weight loss of about 4.2 pounds over a little under four months.[9] Another study found that when people increased their intake of soluble fiber by 10 grams a day, their belly fat decreased by 3.7 percent in five years,[10] while still another showed that soluble fiber can boost the immune system.[11]

So, from now on, you will be eating fiber throughout the day—all five times you eat, in fact. Yes, you might notice that you may need to go to the bathroom more frequently, especially at first, but that's a GOOD thing. The longer food sits in your colon, the more it messes with your blood sugar (and eventually turns to fat). Fiber helps us clear out the intestinal trash that's not doing our bodies any favors.

A Fiber Primer

There are two types of fiber: soluble (meaning it dissolves in water and is digested by your body) and insoluble (meaning it doesn't dissolve in water, and rather than being digested by your body merely passes through, aiding the digestive process). Both soluble fiber (found in seeds, oat bran, lentils, and apples) and insoluble fiber (found in whole grains, vegetables, and beans) are absolutely essential for maintaining good digestion and fighting a huge range of diseases.

Fiber's many health advantages are especially important when it comes to weight loss. Fiber makes us feel fuller longer, which is a key to curbing cravings. When you drink a cup of juice (which has no fiber), your blood sugar spikes and shortly thereafter dips. The result is that, half an hour later, you're already craving yet another cup of juice, an endless supply of still more calories.

This is not the case with fiber-packed blended drinks. Soluble fiber in particular slows the body's absorption of sugar, which steadies the body's insulin levels and prevents those ups and downs that make us so ravenously hungry and lead to such disastrous bingeing. Fiber in beverages, by contrast, can actually make you feel fuller than you would otherwise, a 2010 study found, as fibrous foods continue to expand in your stomach.[12] That is, the more fiber in the food, the less you will need to feel full; a 2009 study found that people who ate an apple before lunch ate 15 percent fewer calories than those who had applesauce or drank apple juice.[13]

Because fiber keeps us satisfied for so much longer, we tend to eat less and so over time, we lose more weight. A recent study has shown that fiber consumption can in fact triple weight loss and make us 62 percent less likely to develop diabetes, while a USDA study found that eating 36 grams of fiber a day can prevent the body from absorbing 130 calories a day.[14] Fiber-rich foods are also more calorically dense than low-fiber foods—that is, high-calorie foods tend to be low in fiber, while low-calorie foods tend to be high in fiber.

Making fiber the centerpiece of your diet is one of the best ways to control your appetite and get more out of every calorie. You'll notice immediately when you start drinking my smoothies that you will NOT feel hungry after you've had one—not five minutes later, and not two hours later, either. A lot of that is thanks to the high amounts of fiber you'll be eating.

4

Breaking Up with Sugar

Thirty years ago, when I started in the fitness industry, conventional wisdom had us believe that fat was the demon. Afterward, salt became the biggest bad guy. More recently, carbs have become public enemy number one. Now that we have far more scientific insight, we know not one of these three is the significant driver of our national health crisis. The main culprit by far has always been sugar.

It sounds like a plot straight out of a spy movie, but the sugar industry has been paying scientists to create studies that point the health finger at fat since at least the late 1960s.[1] This practice is still going strong—in 2015, the *New York Times* reported that Coca-Cola paid scientists to produce studies that painted sugar in a favorable light,[2] and in 2016, the Associated Press published reports that a trade association of candy makers influenced researchers to produce a study that found kids who ate candy tend to weigh less than kids who don't.[3] Seriously, you can't make this stuff up!

As I've always said, any diet will work in the short term to help you lose weight. However, if you want to lose weight *and* truly transform your health, you've got to reduce your consumption of added sugars. Yet that is exactly what most American's *aren't* doing; we are eating way, way too much of the sweet stuff.

In fact, Americans eat more sugar than people in any other country in the world—averaging just over 130 pounds of sugar every year.[4] Compare that to the fact that we ate only about 45 pounds per person per year in 1900, and approximately 75 pounds per person per year in 1950. At this rate, we'll be eating nothing but sugar in another few hundred years![5]

Sugar Consumption around the World

If you look at the world's healthiest countries (according to the World Population Review in 2020[6]), you'll see that the United States comes in a lackluster thirty-fifth. You'll also see that we are eating a lot more sugar per day than those healthiest countries are, and that the more sugar a country eats, generally, the lower down on the list it appears (except for Iceland, which makes up for its sweet tooth with a high level of healthy seafood and seaweed consumption).

Health Ranking	Country	Per Capita Sugar Consumption (teaspoons per day)
1	Spain	20
2	Italy	16.4
3	Iceland	26
4	Japan	16.2
5	Switzerland	21.7
7	Australia	27.3
17	Netherlands	29.2
20	Ireland	27.6
23	Germany	29.4
35	United States of America	36.1

It's not a shocker that we're eating as much sugar as we are: a 2015 study published in the journal the *Lancet Diabetes & Endocrinology* found that 74 percent of American food products contain regular or low-calorie sweeteners.[7] If you're not thinking about what you're eating, and just grabbing food off the shelves according to what sounds good, you're basically going to be having dessert for every meal.

Sugar Wreaks Havoc on Your Body

Why is eating as much sugar as we do so bad for us? We know eating sugar can give us cavities, but you may not realize all the ways it breaks down other parts of your body. Here's a quick tour through the highlights:

Hiding in Plain Sight

The most common sources of added sugars in the American diet are:

Soda

Energy and sport drinks

Fruit juice

Coffee drinks

Candy

Ice cream, gelato, and frozen yogurt

Cookies, cakes, and donuts

Flavored yogurts

Breakfast cereals and granola

But the foods you might not realize also contain significant amounts of sugar include:

Ketchup

Salsa

Barbecue sauce

Salad dressings

Bottled marinades

Bottled ice tea

Pasta sauce

Granola bars

Cereal bars

Protein bars

Frozen meals

Applesauce

Cocktails and cocktail mixers

Tonic water

Lemonade

Gummy fruit snacks

Peanut butter

Nondairy milks

Bread

Beef jerky

Protein powder

• *Sugar and your brain.* The link between sugar consumption and high blood glucose levels is so well established that Alzheimer's is now known as Type 3 diabetes. The inflammation sugar kicks off also affects the brain, contributing to brain fog, difficulty focusing, and ADD and ADHD symptoms. (Yet what do we most often feed our kids? Everything with added sugar—cereals, donuts, flavored yogurts, ice cream, cookies, and cakes. It's not good for us, and it's not good for them, either.)

• *Sugar and inflammation.* Sugar gets broken down into lactic acid, which, as its name suggests, is acidic and therefore corrosive. That corrosion can damage cells throughout your body and trigger an immune response, otherwise known as inflammation. And inflammation is a primary contributor to Alzheimer's, heart disease, cancer, and diabetes.

• *Sugar and immunity.* We've known for decades that eating added sugars impairs immune function. A landmark 1973 study either gave participants sucrose, fructose, glucose, honey, or orange juice; or had them fast. They then drew blood so they could assess immune function. Everyone who got the sugar had a significantly decreased level of phagocytes—immune cells that eat bacteria and other foreign invaders. And the results lasted five hours after eating the sugar. Having a healthy immune system was always important, but since the coronavirus came on the scene in 2020, it's even more important to keep your immunity primed so that it can protect you during this (and the next) pandemic.

• *Sugar and insulin sensitivity.* When you eat sugar, the levels of glucose in your bloodstream rise. Your brain will trigger the release of insulin, which shuttles glucose out of the blood. But when your blood glucose levels stay elevated, because you're eating sugar throughout the day, so do your insulin levels. Eventually, your insulin receptors get burned out and can't hear the messages insulin is sending. This is known as insulin resistance, and it's a precursor to Type 2 diabetes. It's estimated that one in three Americans have insulin resistance.

• *Sugar and sleep.* Sugar and poor sleep are a chicken-or-the-egg situation: if you don't sleep well, you'll be more likely to crave sugary foods the next afternoon because you'll need the quick energy hit; if you eat sugary foods late in the day, it will leave you too stimulated to sleep well. In fact, a 2016 study found that folks who eat more sugar-laden foods sleep less deeply and wake up more frequently than people who eat less.[8] The bottom line is this: eating a lot of added sugar makes it harder to get sleep, and the lack of quality sleep makes it harder to stop eating sugary foods.

• *Sugar and weight gain.* Your body can only use so much glucose. Whatever sugar you eat above this small amount gets stored as fat. In addition, as I mentioned, sugar triggers the release of insulin. What I haven't yet covered is that in addition to shuttling glucose out of the blood so that it can be stored as fat, insulin stimulates the release of the hunger-regulating hormone leptin. When your leptin levels are perpetually high, your cells develop leptin resistance, which means you never feel full. That's when you end up eating a lot of extra calories that you don't really need because you aren't getting the "that's enough" signal. And that contributes to weight gain.

• *Sugar and mental health.* Inflammation plays a role in depression, so when you eat sugar, you create an environment that is conducive to depression. The sensations sugar can give you—such as a high followed by a crash and fuzzy thinking—are also similar to symptoms of anxiety. So, while sugar doesn't cause anxiety per se, it can exacerbate it. Finally, sugar is extremely addictive, which means it can make you irritable and rash when you don't have it.

• *Sugar and cancer.* Cancer cells rely on glucose for fuel. And not just a little bit of sugar; according to WebMD, a cancer cell requires 200 times more sugar to generate the same amount of energy as a healthy cell.[9] That's not to say sugar *causes* cancer, although there is evidence to suggest a direct link, but that cancer needs sugar to grow unchecked. Think about that the next time you want to scarf down a bag of peach gummy rings!

Not All Sugar Is Created Equal

There are many different kinds of sugar, but in my mind they fall into two groups: obvious (found in typical sweets like cookies, candy, cakes, and soda) and hidden. These are the sugars that are hiding in places we would never expect—like tomato sauce—and in foods and drinks we think are pretty healthy, like energy drinks, granola, trail mix, and dried fruit. It's one thing to decide not to have the obvious sugars, to get the ice cream out of your freezer and the candy out of your desk drawer. It's something to celebrate. But if you don't also address the hidden sugars, it can really add up and sabotage your efforts to be healthy—and you may not even realize it's happening.

It is vital that you start to read labels and look for the grams of added sugars—those are any form of sugar that isn't found in the whole version of the food. As I've already covered, fruit juice, for example, contains natural sugar, but not in a natural form because the juice has been removed from the fiber, protein, vitamins, and minerals that are found in the whole fruit and that help mitigate the impact on your blood sugar. When you eat dried fruit, you can get up to ten times the amount of sugar in the whole version of the fruit in one serving, because without the water contained in the grape, the raisin is basically just a very densely packed sugar delivery system.

Beyond avoiding obvious and hidden added sugars, you can make your journey to living a low-added-sugar life by ensuring you eat the right mix of fiber, protein, fat, and carbs at every meal and have sustaining snacks during the day so that you avoid a blood sugar dip and do not fall prey to sugar cravings.

Sneaky Names for **Sugar**

Food manufacturers use more than fifty different names for sugar in an attempt to sneak sweeteners in under the radar, but your body doesn't care what name sugar is called. That's why it's important to become an educated reader of labels—even on foods you consider to be healthy. Keep your eye out for any of these ingredients, and remember they mean "added sugar."

Agave nectar/syrup

Barley malt (syrup)

Beet sugar

Blackstrap molasses

Buttered syrup

Brown rice syrup

Cane juice (crystals)

Caramel

Carob syrup

Coconut sugar

Corn sweetener

Corn syrup (solids)

Crystalline fructose

Dehydrated cane juice

Dextrin

Diastatic malt

Evaporated cane juice

Ethyl maltol

Florida crystals

Fructose

Fruit juice (concentrate)

Galactose

Glucose (syrup) (solids)

Golden syrup

High-fructose corn syrup

Honey

Lactose

Malt syrup

Maltodextrin

Maltola

Mannose

Maple syrup

Molasses

Muscovado

Panocha

Refiner's syrup

Rice syrup

Saccharose

Sorghum syrup

Sucanat

Sucrose

Sweet sorghum

Syrup

Treacle

Turbinado sugar

Alternative Sweeteners Are Still Sugar

There's a misconception that a natural sugar—such as honey or maple syrup—is better for you than one that's more processed, such as table sugar. While there are some subtle differences in how much and how quickly each sweetener will raise your blood sugar levels, no added sugar is "good" for you.

One helpful tool for keeping tabs on your sugar intake is the glycemic index, which is just a numeric way of rating the impact a particular carbohydrate-containing food has on your blood sugar levels. In general, the more fat, protein, and/or fiber a food has, the longer it will take to be digested and the smaller the resulting rise in blood sugar.

As you can see from the box on the right, there are some forms of sugar that are lower on the glycemic index than others. But again, your body doesn't care what type of sugar it is called. Even though honey ranks lower on the glycemic index than table sugar, it still triggers a spike in blood glucose that wouldn't happen if you skipped the sweetener altogether. That blood sugar spike still cues the release of insulin, which then lowers your blood sugar levels quickly, leading to an energy crash that then triggers a craving for more carbs.

Another important piece of being able to go without added sugar is retraining your palate to appreciate less sweet foods, and even the lowest glycemic-index sweetener doesn't help you do that.

The good news is that as you move through the Body Reset Diet, your cravings for sugar will abate, because you'll be eating plenty of fiber, protein, and healthy fat so that you won't be as prone to the blood sugar spikes and resulting crashes that cause sugar cravings. Also, once you're done with the three phases and have moved on to maintenance, you'll be able to reintroduce treats that use added sugar as part of your two free meals a week.

GLYCEMIC INDEX OF VARIOUS SUGARS

Sugar	Glycemic index
Glucose (corn syrup)	100
Rice syrup	98
Sucrose (table sugar)	65
Blackstrap molasses	55
Maple syrup	54
Honey	50
Lactose (the sugar in dairy)	46
Medjool dates	42
Coconut sugar	35
Palm sugar	35
Xylitol	12
Erythritol (a sugar alcohol)	0

The Only Kind of Sugar That's Okay during the Body Reset

It's true that fruit has natural sugar in it, and as a result, so do the smoothies on the Body Reset Diet. It's important to note that the natural sugars in fruit come packaged with protein, fiber, and in some cases fat (such as avocado or coconut), and that these other nutrients blunt the impact of the natural sugars on your blood sugar levels.

It's no accident that I have you drinking two fruit-based smoothies a day in Phase I of the Body Reset Diet: it's to help you wean yourself off sugar without going into total withdrawal. Remember, most Americans are eating 17 teaspoons of sugar a day. Having plenty of fruit through your two fruit-based smoothies a day in Phase I, and then tapering that down through the other two phases, helps you wean off sugar slowly so that you don't feel out of sorts or experience cravings that are all but impossible to resist.

If you're really struggling with sugar cravings at any point during the Body Reset Diet, I feel your pain. I had a sugar addiction for years. First, I kept my sugar consumption a secret because I have two brothers with diabetes, and I didn't want them to see me eating what they couldn't have. As an adult, I was a personal trainer and it felt too out of alignment to be loud and proud about my daily pastries or cookies (or oftentimes, both). Basically, I was a huge hypocrite. It wasn't until my wife came to me with our credit card bill and asked why I was spending $250 a month at the coffee shop that I was forced to reckon with my sugar dependence. The bill was that high because I was getting a coffee *and* a cookie *and* a scone, almost every day. She was laughing about it, but I almost cried when I saw the definitive evidence that I was addicted. Everything else in my life was so healthy—I was having nutritious whole foods for breakfast, lunch, and dinner, I walked 14,000 steps a day, I slept well. Sugar was my last vice.

To help myself, and to help others who were in the same boat, I created a product called Sweetkick that has two parts: a daily fiber powder that keeps you feeling full, regulates your blood sugar levels, and helps ward off cravings; and a breath mint made from three plants that blocks your tongue from tasting anything sweet. You drink the powder in the morning to start you off on the right foot, and then you eat a mint after each meal so you can't taste any of the sweet things that you might otherwise habitually reach for. You may still buy the scone and take a bite, but you won't be able to get that hit of sugar bliss. It helps you see those "treats" for what they really are—empty calories. I am not trying to push the product in this book, but I do want you to know that if cutting out added sugars is making you quake in your boots, there is something that can help. (Visit sweetkick.com for more information.)

One note: After you've completed all three phases and are in the maintenance mode, there are no rules or even guidelines about your two free meals a week. If the thought of never eating any sugary treats the rest of your life is scaring you away, know that you can have them twice a week on the Body Reset Diet as part of your free meal. As long as you can keep it to that minimal frequency (meaning, if you have a little you can stop yourself from having a lot more), it won't impact your weight or your health.

II

The First 15 Days
of the Rest
of Your Life

5

An Overview of the Body Reset Diet

All right, so let's get down to it. First off, as I've already mentioned, throughout these initial 15 days you'll get into the habit of eating five times daily to maximize the efficiency of your metabolism. Five categories of ingredients, five minutes of prep time, five meals daily—that's my highly successful formula.

During the first five days of the Body Reset Diet, I've even further simplified both the categories of ingredients and the time it takes to make a meal out of them. With the help of a blender, you can make a whole meal in 2 minutes flat, including all prep time. I promise you, there is NO easier way to make amazingly delicious and good-for-you meals, to enjoy either at home or on the go.

Whether you're having a smoothie or a blended soup, a solid meal or a snack, you will always be eating five times a day, at intervals timed to keep your blood sugar stable and your metabolism at its most efficient.

The Three Phases

The Body Reset Diet is broken into three distinct 5-day phases lasting a total of 15 days. You'll be alternating nutritious, delicious, and filling smoothies and blended soups with a number of snacks and meals, all of which you can toss together in 5 minutes, max.

Harley's **Reset** Template

You'll:

- Eat five times a day to rev up your metabolism.

- Follow specific nutritional criteria for each meal.

- Build each meal around the same categories of ingredients.

- Prepare each meal in 5 minutes or less.

After you complete the 15-day kick-start, you will follow a much looser long-term version of this plan. By this point, you'll have learned the benefits of:

- Eating five times a day.
- Moving consistently from morning till night.
- Preparing your own meals.

You will also be looking and feeling so good that you'll be motivated to continue this plan on your own. But for the first 15 days, I'm going to hold your hand and tell you exactly what you have to do and why you need to do it.

PHASE I

Diet: In Phase I, between Days 1 and 5, you'll be drinking two smoothies and one blended soup a day and eating two snacks. This period will be the greatest adjustment for your body and brain, but don't worry; this is the reset portion of the Body Reset. The meals are high volume, which means that you'll feel like you are eating a lot of food throughout the entire plan.

Movement: During these first few days, you'll give up your spin class or boot camp and simply walk—a minimum of 10,000 steps a day, a very achievable goal you can track with the help of an activity tracker, a tiny device that counts the number of steps you take a day. (Trust me—it will become your favorite new toy! See page 102 for tips on picking out the perfect one.)

PHASE II

Diet: By Phase II, between Days 6 and 10, you'll still be eating five times a day, providing your body with a steady supply of fuel, but now you'll be drinking only two blended meals (whether a fruit-based smoothie or veggie-based soup) and having one solid—nonblended, but still healthy, delicious, and extremely easy to prepare—meal a day, plus your usual choice of snacks between the meals.

Movement: In Phase II, you're going to bump your minimum daily steps up to 12,000 a day. Don't get too nervous about this—that's really only about 10 more minutes of walking at a normal pace. You'll also begin a super-simple 5-minute at-home fitness routine three days a week to tone your changing body. These exercises will be extremely easy to do and require no equipment, and I'll offer a variety of modifications to suit different fitness levels.

PHASE III

Diet: In Phase III, you'll have just one smoothie or blended soup a day, plus two meals and two snacks.

Movement: Continue to walk throughout your day until you've logged 12,000 steps. Your strengthening routine will be a slightly extended version of the super-simple resistance exercises I introduced in Phase II. In addition to keeping up your regular walking, you'll be alternating between two 5-minute circuits of resistance training five days a week. You can do these simple exercises in any room in your house, and with little to no equipment.

	Phase I (5 Days)	Phase II (5 Days)	Phase III (5 Days and Beyond)
Breakfast	Smoothie	Smoothie	Smoothie
Snack 1	Snack	Snack	Snack
Lunch	Smoothie	Smoothie or blended soup	Meal
Snack 2	Snack	Snack	Snack
Dinner	Blended soup	Meal	Meal

THE REST OF YOUR LIFE

Diet: You'll still be eating five times a day, but in combinations that you design yourself. You'll have one smoothie or blended soup a day, two snacks, and two solid meals. And twice a week you can enjoy "free meals," when you hit the town (or fridge) and eat whatever you want.

Movement: Keep up with the 12,000 steps a day! This I want you to do seven days a week, 365 days a year, for the rest of your life. This simple modification to your daily habits will transform you from a couch potato to a fit, energetic person—and all you have to do is walk. Five days a week, you'll be doing a slightly increased version of your A and B resistance-training circuits for a total of 10 minutes a day, or less than an hour a week (i.e., less time than you used to spend on a single grueling spin class).

So there's your cheat sheet—sound pretty simple and straightforward? Trust me, it is.

"When I was at my heaviest, I thought that I was as comfortable as possible because I gave into every bad craving and let myself rest and relax whenever I wanted to. 'I deserve it,' I told myself. Adjusting to exercise and clean eating was a challenge at first, but as I embraced the uncomfortable and the weight fell off, I felt more alive than I ever have in my whole life. My eyes brightened, my skin got clearer, I slept better, I had enough energy to bounce off the walls, and I had a better sense of structure and discipline to be more productive. I feel healthy now and it's the sexiest, most comfortable feeling ever! And I deserve it!"

—CHERIE N., LOST 9 POUNDS IN 15 DAYS

PHASE

6

Getting Started

Phase I: What You'll Be Doing

You will be eating five times a day: two smoothies, one blended soup, and two snacks. You will be walking a minimum of 10,000 steps per day (for easy ways of achieving this goal, see page 104).

What You'll Need
- A blender (see page 31)
- An activity tracker (see page 102)
- A shopping list (see page 84)

ASSEMBLING THE SMOOTHIES AND BLENDED SOUPS

The more you know about what's going into your smoothies and blended soups, the more confident you'll be about substituting similar ingredients from the same categories to add more variety to your drinks later on. First, you need to know that when I say "smoothie" I am NOT talking about those sugar bombs you get from "healthy" smoothie counters at the food court. Most of those overpriced concoctions add untold hundreds of calories to your daily intake with a through-the-roof sugar content that will send your appetite spiraling into overdrive.

The Body Reset Diet smoothies won't leave you with a massive sugar hangover nor do they taste excessively "healthy." In smoothie making, as in so many other aspects of modern life, the pendulum keeps swinging between two extremes: we're either drinking sherbet-stuffed smoothies with 1,800 calories per serving or we're blending jugs of bok choy and red onion for breakfast. I'm sorry, but that's gross. You do NOT have to chug disgusting vegetable-only medleys to lose weight. Food is one of the great pleasures in life, and it should remain so even while you are slimming down.

Forget about both sugary drinks and the kale-stuffed elixirs. This is not a zero-sum game: the Body Reset Diet smoothies are good for your body and they taste amazing. The same goes for the blended soups—the soups I've created for you are as easy to make as the smoothies—and as tasty. It's just that they have a more savory taste profile than the smoothies, and they help you load up on veggies—a category of food most Americans eat way too little of, which is a crying shame because vegetables are amazing nutrient-delivery systems. In addition to vitamins and minerals, vegetables are a great source of fiber, healthy carbs, and, yes, even some protein (½ cup of cooked spinach has 3 grams, and 1 cup

Components of the
Perfect Smoothie

- Liquid base (milk, dairy or nondairy; water or flavored water)
- Lean protein (plain nonfat Greek yogurt, protein powder, peanut butter, tofu)
- Healthy fat (nuts, seeds, avocado)
- High-fiber carbohydrate (pretty much any fruit or vegetable you can name, though some are better than others; see page 71)

You'll notice that a number of these ingredients overlap—for example, the milk used as the liquid base is also a source of protein, and healthy fats like avocados are also fruits (yes, technically, they are fruit—a berry, to be exact).

That's why all those stringent (and to my mind ridiculous) food-combining diets—in which you can never eat a carbohydrate at the same meal as a fat, for example—make absolutely no sense to me. Bean-based diets are incredibly healthy, and the nutritional profile of a bean is equal parts carbohydrate, fiber, and fat. And let me tell you, this nation is not getting fat from eating too many kidney beans!

The key is variety, consuming the widest possible range of foods every time you sit down to eat. My smoothie and blended soup recipes take all the guesswork out of this balancing act by offering everything you need in one delicious drink.

The Case for **Milk**

Dairy products have gotten a bad rap in the past few years, mostly because of environmental enthusiasts (who are concerned about the impact of dairy farming on the environment) and misinformation about the antibiotics and hormones in it. As with so much of the health "wisdom" we're force-fed, this is nonsense—milk products are among the healthiest foods you can eat!

It's important to know that the government regulates the dairy industry more stringently than almost any other food sector. If a dairy farm has even trace amounts of antibiotics in their milk, the entire truckload is dumped. If the farm is caught three times with traces of antibiotics, they are shut down. It's a very high standard that they're held to.

I'm sure you've heard some well-meaning "expert" argue that humans are the only species that drinks milk from another animal—well, so what? We've been doing it for thousands of years. We're also the only species who can fly airplanes and write sonnets and solve physics equations.

Rich in protein, calcium, vitamin D, phosphorus, and other nutrients that have been proven to build your bones and teeth, as well as promote the healthy function of your muscles and blood vessels, milk is one of the most perfect foods for the human body. Calcium can help the body switch from fat-storing to fat-burning mode, keeping you slim.

High-calcium foods like milk and yogurt can also directly aid weight-loss efforts. Researchers at the University of Knoxville have found that high-calcium foods, notably dairy sources, have been shown to increase the rate of body-fat breakdown and preserve metabolism during dieting.[1] One 2012 study found that an ingredient in milk can protect against obesity, while another concluded that dairy-rich products can help people shed belly fat.[2] And there's still more evidence: a 2019 study found that overweight women who ate multiple servings of low-fat dairy a day—four or five—lost on average 4 percent of total body weight and 3 percent of body fat—significantly more than participants who merely took a calcium and vitamin D supplement (two nutrients provided by dairy) or who took a placebo.[3]

It's no coincidence that some of the healthiest countries in the world have made dairy products a dietary staple. When I was researching my previous book, *The 5-Factor World Diet,* I was pleased (but not at all surprised) to learn that several of the healthiest countries in the world have dairy-based diets. Svelte Scandinavians often drink a glass of milk with meals, and the French and Greeks both regularly eat yogurt, a fantastic source of the active probiotic cultures we need to keep our immune systems up and running. Many of the smoothies in this book contain Greek yogurt for that very reason—and because it's satisfying and delicious.

As with everything in life, though, not all dairy products have the same nutritional properties. A nonfat plain Greek yogurt will obviously have a different effect on your body than a hunk of Cheddar cheese, precisely because these are extremely different foods that we shouldn't lump together indiscriminately. Because the fat that's in dairy isn't as heart-healthy as fats from vegetables or fish, we'll be sticking with nonfat or low-fat milk products in our drinks, which give us essential nutrients while still leaving room, calorically speaking, for fats from better sources, such as nuts, seeds, and avocados. And while I don't expect you to replace all your groceries with organic substitutions, I would recommend buying at least hormone-free dairy products whenever possible, since the United States is one of the few countries that still permit dairy farmers to use the scary recombinant bovine growth hormone (rBGH) or recombinant bovine somatotropin (rBST) in cows. If you buy organic dairy, in addition to being hormone-free it will be free of pesticides and antibiotics.

of raw broccoli has 2.6 grams!). It's my hope that by swapping out one of the fruit-based smoothies a day for a veggie-heavy blended soup, you'll see how easy and delicious it is to eat more vegetables without having to mow your way through a huge salad twice a day. You'll also get a chance to wean yourself off having a sweet taste at every meal—and because the soups have the right blend of fiber, protein, carbs, and fat, you'll still feel plenty full.

Both the smoothies and the blended soups will help stabilize your blood sugar and curb those all-too-familiar hunger pangs, and they're so satisfying precisely because they all contain the right combination of foods in the right proportions.

And about that. Once you understand the science behind the ingredients, you'll be able to create an infinite variety of these delicious beverages whenever you want—depending on what's in season or just what mood you're in. Losing weight means combining the right kinds of foods every time you eat. To meet my criteria for a complete meal—one that delivers all the nutrients you need and keeps you craving free until it's time to eat again—each smoothie and blended soup must contain several predetermined categories of ingredients in addition to the base: a lean protein, a healthy fat, and a high-fiber carbohydrate.

Ingredient Category #1: Liquid Base

The liquid is the first ingredient you place into the blender when making a smoothie or a blended soup. (A tip for optimal blending is to start with the light ingredients and proceed to the heavier ones, though there are no hard-and-fast rules—experiment as you go and figure out what works for you.)

My smoothies generally use either milk or water as a base, and my blended soups start with water. A lot of people ask me about substituting almond milk or oat milk. I know some people like to avoid cow's milk for philosophical reasons or have a legitimate allergy to dairy, and

I support that 100 percent; in that case, just make sure the nondairy milk you use for your smoothie base is unsweetened. However, I don't think the health promises of nut milks equal the nutrients that cow's milk provides. If you were to make almond milk or oat milk at home, you'd soak the almonds or the oats overnight in water. The next day you'd blend that mixture, then filter out all the solids. There's very little almond or oat in what's left, and that's when you make it at home and can control all the variables. Commercial nondairy milks, whether they're almond, rice, soy, or oat, add a bunch of gums, stabilizers, and flavorings. To my mind, they're just not worth it.

Remember, it's all about making every calorie count, so stick to the simplest liquids to get your smoothie started—and that generally means milk or water. If it's a white smoothie that calls for milk as a base, make it either nonfat, 1 percent fat, or 2 percent fat, depending on your taste. Because we want every calorie to count, whole milk just has too many calories from fat, and as I said earlier, milk fat is not a high-quality fat. When you choose nonfat, 1 percent, or 2 percent milk, those calories are more protein-based than fat-based, which will help make sure you get enough of ingredient category #2.

Ingredient Category #2: Lean Protein

Major rule to live by: We need to consume protein *every single time* we eat because it helps us feel full. Forget about a plate of pasta and tomato sauce—that doesn't count as a meal because it doesn't contain adequate protein, one of the three macronutrients used as building blocks of our bodies. High-quality animal sources of protein include chicken, fish, meat, eggs, and dairy; vegetarian sources include whole grains like quinoa and brown rice, legumes like beans and lentils, soy products like tofu, and nuts (while nuts do contain some protein, they are primarily a fat—anywhere from 83 to 93 percent of their calories come from fat). The one issue I have with all the vegetarian sources of protein is that their protein content is secondary or tertiary to other nutrients in the food. For example, while brown rice contains a small amount of protein, it's still 95 percent carbohydrate. And while nuts contain protein, they're still anywhere between 80 to 90 percent fat. So the challenge if you're using a vegetarian option as your protein source is to use copious amounts, and in the process you'll end up ingesting much higher amounts of carbohydrates and fats than you might otherwise want or need.

We need protein for numerous reasons. First, unlike carbohydrates or fat, we can't store protein as fat; we must either use it or excrete it, which is why people who eat protein at every meal consistently lose more weight than people who don't. Loading up on protein at breakfast in particular has been shown to be especially effective at reducing food cravings and overeating later in the day.[4]

Protein is also critical for maintaining muscle tissue; a 2011 study of postmenopausal women on diets found that eating protein throughout the day helped them preserve muscle even as they lost fat—exactly what we're trying to do here![5] Another study confirmed the weight-loss attributes of a high-protein diet, finding that the consumption of protein increases both satiety and the retention of lean muscle mass.[6]

And remember, the more lean muscle tissue you have, the more calories you'll burn throughout the day and night, independent of any physical activity. Just getting enough protein in your diet can help moderate your intake of food and keep obesity at bay.[7] Protein also is important for regulating your resting metabolism (the amount of calories we burn at rest), and it contributes to a feeling of fullness, which is important for curbing hunger between meals. As an added benefit, a 2016 study found that overweight participants who increased their protein intake while trying to lose weight also enjoyed improved sleep quality—and since sleep is such a foundational component of health, eating more protein is a way that following the

Body Reset Diet can help improve your overall wellness in a significant way.[8]

Ingredient Category #3: Healthy Fat

Some diet books will tell you to shun all fats if you want to lose weight, but in reality it's not healthy to eliminate fat from our diets altogether. Many others, particularly those espousing a keto diet, will tell you to make the vast majority of your calories come from fat. While fat is essential, good nutrition is all about balance, and if you eat that many calories from fat you'll either (a) not get enough carbs and protein, or (b) still get plenty of carbs and protein, but consume so many extra calories that you gain weight. Neither of these options is what we're after.

Fat is, along with protein and carbohydrates, one of the three categories of macronutrients that our bodies need to function. Fat's a major source of energy and a big element in satiety that helps the body absorb vitamins A, D, E, and K. Fat is important for our hormones, nerves, reproductive system, and skin. Our brains need fat, too, especially omega-3 and omega-6 fatty acids, which we can get only through food; the body does not produce these essential nutrients on its own. Most of us get too many omega-6s and not enough omega-3s, so we need to make an effort to reverse that imbalance by favoring omega-3–rich fats, in particular.

But though fats are essential, they're not all equally beneficial. There are good fats and bad fats, and we should optimize the levels of "healthy" fats in our diet like those in avocados and almonds while steering clear of the bad fats—namely, saturated fats (most of which come from animal sources and trans fats, which are found in processed foods and hydrogenated oils). When we reduce saturated fats, entirely cut out trans fats, and up our intake of monounsaturated fats (found in nuts and vegetable oils) and polyunsaturated fatty acids (derived from vegetable sources and fish), we'll be well on our way to getting the body of our dreams—and that's exactly what the Body Reset Diet guides you to do.

BAD FATS are broken into two big categories: saturated fats and trans fats. Both saturated fats and trans fats can raise "bad" and lower "good" cholesterol levels, and have been linked to heart disease. Saturated fats are mostly found in animal products like red meat, poultry skin, whole milk, butter, and egg yolks, though some vegetable sources such as coconut oil, palm oil, and palm kernel oil also contain high levels. Trans fats, or hydrogenated fats, are for the most part artificial—they're predominantly found in commercially processed food products like doughnuts, cookies, and fried foods—and have zero redeeming qualities. While eating small amounts of saturated fats is unavoidable in most diets, there's absolutely no reason why you should be eating trans fats, period.

GOOD FATS—the fats that you will be eating while on the Body Reset Diet—shouldn't raise total cholesterol. They actually lower our LDL (bad cholesterol) while raising our HDL (good cholesterol). We absolutely must include these good fats as part of a healthy diet. Like the bad fats, the good fats can be grouped into several categories. Monounsaturated fats are found in nuts, avocados, and various vegetable oils, particularly olive oil, which consists of approximately 75 percent monounsaturated fats.

Also critical, especially for brain health, are those polyunsaturated fats found in various fish and vegetable sources, such as flaxseed and chia seeds. Polyunsaturated fats are essential because they provide our bodies with omega-3 fatty acids (or, in the case of the seeds, the omega-3 precursor alpha-linolenic acid, which the body must convert to omega-3). These "good fats" can even help fight Alzheimer's disease and prevent the brain from shrinking.[9] And healthy fats can also improve our skin, hair, nails, and overall appearance. If you eat better, you look better—it's as simple as that.

Ingredient Category #4: High-Fiber Carbohydrates

Though they've gotten a bad rap in recent years, carbohydrates are not at all bad for you. On the contrary, they're one of the most important parts of a healthy diet, and studies show that people who consume at least 50 percent of their calories from carbohydrates are *least* likely to be obese.[10] But as with all foods, there are good carbohydrates and bad carbohydrates, and to lose weight you must understand the difference.

The healthiest carbohydrates—the ones you want to build your diet around—are the ones that rank relatively low on the glycemic index (GI), which is a system that measures the rate at which our blood sugar rises in response to eating certain foods. High-GI foods—like white flour–based breads and pastas or sugary foods (whether those sugars are natural, as in grapes, or less natural, as in licorice)—cause an instant spike in your blood sugar and also in your body's production of insulin. Chronically high levels of insulin are associated with Type 2 diabetes, obesity, and even heart disease. Minimizing your sugar intake is absolutely central to losing weight, and not just because of all the calories sugar contains. It's much wiser to choose low-GI carbohydrates that break down slowly, release energy steadily throughout the day, and take much longer to digest.

We also want carbohydrates with a higher fiber content—that crucial ingredient missing not only from juice but also from the white breads and pastas we wolf down with such abandon. Numerous studies have shown that diets high in fiber can achieve weight loss, and the best all-over source of fiber is fruits and vegetables, which not only lower the risk for certain cancers, stroke, heart disease, and high blood pressure but also help keep the weight off.[11]

What Else You'll Be Eating

I understand that monotony is the death of many diets—and that texture is an important part of our enjoyment of food—so you'll have two snacks a day even in the first phase of the plan. These snacks are all easily accessible, portable, and require limited preparation. I call these snacks C-snacks for a couple of reasons. First, they're for the most part CRUNCHY, which satisfies the very normal desire to chew. Second, C can also stand for CUT, as in cut veggies (everything from celery and carrots to broccoli and zucchini) or fruit. Not all fruit will do, though. Stick to fruit with either edible skin (except grapes) or edible seeds (like berries) or to citrus fruits.

Now, don't get me wrong, I'm not saying that all other fruits are bad for you—not at all. All fruits are good for you, with the nutrients and enzymes our bodies need to flourish—and that's why I include such a wide range of them in the smoothie recipes. However, if you're trying to lose weight fast, stick to the healthier fruits with less sugar and more fiber that will promote faster weight loss in the first 15 days.

SNACK FRUITS

Eat More...		Than...	
Apples	Berries	Mangoes	Cantaloupes
Pears	Cherries	Papayas	Honeydew melons
Peaches	Kiwifruit	Bananas	Watermelons
Nectarines	Oranges	Grapes	
Plums		Pineapples	

You can also eat CRACKERS with a high fiber content; check the label and make sure there are at least 5 grams of fiber and less than 5 grams of sugar per 100 calories. Some of my favorite brands are Finn Crisp, Ryvita, Wasa, and Kavli.

Another major detail about these snacks: As with any meal, they

MUST be eaten with a protein! Fruit alone is not enough. Carrots on their own might be "healthy," but they are not a complete snack. Quite often, eating these alone can make you even hungrier.

This is nonnegotiable, because a meal is not a meal and a snack is not a snack unless there's protein and fiber involved, so *every* time you sit down to eat make sure you include both. That means crackers on their own aren't enough; you must combine them with a dip (made from nonfat Greek yogurt seasoned with onion soup or ranch mix) or maybe some hummus or a low-fat bean dip.

All the snacks should be about 150 calories and contain at least 5 grams of fiber, 5 grams of protein, and *less* than 10 grams of sugar.

A few examples of some easy combinations you can try:[†]

- Celery with almond butter
- Whole-grain crackers with hummus
- Carrots with onion dip (made from nonfat Greek yogurt and onion soup mix)

[†] *Snack bars, cereals, and other prepackaged snacks must meet the basic nutritional requirements of the rest of your C-snacks: They must have no more than 150 calories and contain at least 5 grams of fiber, 5 grams of protein, and less than 10 grams of sugar.*

Popcorn

It's a great idea to keep some low-fat popcorn around the house for a delicious snack in a hurry. My favorite brand is Naked: a 150-calorie serving contains approximately 6 grams of fiber, 5 grams of protein, and 4 grams of fat. The Whole Foods 365 brand is also a great low-fat popcorn, and there are several other good microwaveable varieties as well. Of course, if you really want to make a habit of eating this healthy snack, I suggest you buy an air popper for about $15 and just pop whole kernels. The popcorn tastes fresher, and your machine will pay for itself in just a few months.

- Low-fat popcorn**†

- Roasted soy nuts**

- Low added-sugar, high-protein, high-fiber snack bars**†

- Freeze-dried green peas (try the ones sold under Target's Archer Farms label)

- Chickpea snacks**† (I like the ones made by Good Bean)

- Apple with low-fat cheese

- Apple with peanut butter

- Pear and sliced lean turkey

- Cucumber and smoked salmon

- Crackers and almond butter

- High-protein, high-fiber cereal (e.g., Kashi Go Lean, Optimum Blueberry Cinnamon)**†

- Steamed edamame**

- A palmful of nuts

- Chia pudding

** *These foods already contain both fiber and protein so they can be eaten as stand-alone snacks.*

† *Snack bars, cereals, and other prepackaged snacks must meet the basic nutritional requirements of the rest of your C-snacks: They must have no more than 150 calories and contain at least 5 grams of fiber, 5 grams of protein, and less than 10 grams of sugar.*

For serving sizes, nutrition information, recommended brands and products, and a more comprehensive list of snacks, see page 213.

What Else You'll Be Drinking

In addition to the smoothies and soups, you need to drink a steady supply of other liquids throughout the day. Water in particular helps you flush out toxins from your body that might be dragging you down and keeping your weight higher than it needs to be.

Drinking helps fill you up and increases satiety, and keeping enough liquid in your body is essential for staying in good shape. Dehydration brings bad side effects, including fatigue, headaches, and muscle cramping, and can very easily be mistaken for hunger. So, the next time you think you're hungry, have a tall glass of water first, and your growling stomach just might quiet down.

For the duration of the Body Reset Diet (and, come to think of it, for the duration of your time on earth), I want you to be drinking *3 to 4 liters of fluids a day,* which might sound like a lot, but trust me, your body will soon grow to love it. Drinking lots of liquids keeps your body clean and detoxed, and it tricks your stomach into feeling fuller than it actually is.

ACCEPTABLE BEVERAGES
Water

The mother of all drinks is water, and I want you to be getting a lot of it every day—around 3 liters if you're a woman and 4 liters if you're a man. And yes, that's a suggested *minimum.* There are lots of different ways you can get your fill of water:

Flat water: My favorite brand of bottled water is PROPEL, but regular tap water always does the trick. You can also invest in a water filter like those made by Brita or PUR for your home.

Sparkling water: You can buy sparkling water like San Pellegrino or Perrier, or you can make your own at home with a Sodastream soda maker (www.sodastreamusa.com), which costs as little as $80 and can save you big bucks in the long term.

Flavored ice cubes or flavored water: If you want to add some subtle flavor to either still or sparkling water, try making flavored ice cubes. To do this, just place the grated peel of an orange or lemon in an ice cube tray and add water. Put the tray in the freezer. A few hours later, add a few flavored ice cubes to your water for a delicious twist.

You can also add a wedge of fruit or a cucumber slice directly to your water.

Coffee/Coffee Drinks

I am a huge fan of caffeine, and in fact I spent three years as a caffeine scientist for the Canadian Department of National Defense, so I know what I'm talking about when I say caffeine can be a great addition to your diet. As long as you aren't adding any caloric sweeteners or full-fat dairy to your coffee, which is naturally calorie free, I encourage you to keep drinking and enjoying your favorite caffeinated beverages. In fact, I don't understand why diet books ever advise otherwise. So many cleanses have you remove all caffeinated beverages from your diet, but why? Caffeine is a proven appetite suppressant and it provides much-

What about
Coconut Water?

Since the first edition of *The Body Reset Diet* came out, I've had a lot of people ask me if they can use coconut water as a base in their smoothies. To me that answer is a clear NO. Coconut water is similar to fruit juice, with slightly less sugar. It may seem as if it's a lot lower in sugar than fruit juice—a cup of coconut water has about 6 grams of sugar, versus 23 grams of sugar in a cup of fruit juice. But if you look closely at the label on a container of coconut water, you'll typically see that there are two or even three servings in there. It's just too easy to get too much sugar.

needed energy, so why would you ever eliminate your morning coffee when it's both good for you and completely delicious?

Coffee in particular contains powerful antioxidants that might prevent the development of Type 2 diabetes and reduce risk factors associated with heart disease and strokes.[12] Coffee drinking could reduce our risk of developing both endometrial and skin cancers, and frequent coffee consumption has been linked to lower rates of Parkinson's disease and Alzheimer's disease.[13] Even decaf can sharpen our memories and lower our chance of developing diabetes.[14] And a 2012 study found that coffee drinkers live longer than everyone else.[15] Maybe that's because researchers have found an association between regular coffee consumption and lower risks of colon cancer,[16] prostate cancer,[17] heart failure, and stroke.[18] So, drink up—provided you skip all the nasty additives we've become so fond of dumping in our coffees. Stick with black coffee or espresso.

Coffee is also a great source of energy. To keep the weight off, we need to get moving (which is much easier said than done when we're laid low by another caffeine-withdrawal migraine—thanks, but no thanks). Of course, as in all things, moderation is key. Too much caffeine can keep you awake, and multiple studies have shown that chronic sleep deprivation makes you fatter. So drink enough caffeine to keep you going—but not too late so that it keeps you awake all night.

Tea

Tea is another deliciously versatile beverage that can be an indispensable diet aid. It's the second most popular drink in the world, outpaced only by water. And though many Americans drink tea regularly, they all too often dump large quantities of sweeteners in it. The same old story . . .

But in its purest form, tea is naturally calorie free. Though all teas come from the same source, different processing methods have produced a range of different varieties, all of which contain different quantities of caffeine and have slightly different health properties. Here are a few things they all have in common: They improve brain health[19] and reduce risk of heart disease, which helps us live longer.[20] They might help us lose weight. A 2010 study out of Kobe University in Japan found that regular consumption of tea can counteract the fattening effect of junk food.[21] A 2019 animal study suggests that tea might protect against weight gain by improving gut health and contributing to a stronger population of beneficial gut bacteria.[22] So, don't be afraid to sip your way through the day.

Experiment with the whole range of teas and find the one you like:

Black tea, which has the most caffeine (though still less than coffee), contains antioxidants known as polyphenols and has weight-loss properties. An exciting area of scientific research that has evolved since I first wrote *The Body Reset Diet* is epigenetics—or the science of how different genes get turned on and turned off. A 2019 study found that black tea beneficially affected the epigenetics of women's genes related to estrogen metabolism and cancer, suggesting that it supports your body all the way down to your DNA.[23]

Green tea and **white tea**, both of which have less caffeine than black and oolong teas, have extremely powerful antioxidant properties that can protect against cancer and heart disease, and both teas can also lower bad cholesterol levels. Green tea in particular might also be a useful weight-loss aid. It's been shown to stabilize blood sugar and reduce people's risk of developing Type 2 diabetes. In one study, diabetic rats given green tea lost significantly more weight and had much lower cholesterol levels than those not treated with the tea.[24] Another study, from 2012 on mice, found that even in conjunction with a high-fat diet green tea can help keep off the pounds.[25]

Oolong tea, a type of green tea, slightly lower on the caffeine scale, is chock-full of polyphenols and catechins, antioxidants renowned for their anti-inflammatory qualities. Oolong tea might also help regulate blood sugar and increase metabolism by 10 percent for two hours after drinking. Several studies found that oolong tea might be an effective obesity treatment, and that regular consumption of oolong tea can lead to weight loss and an improved metabolism.[26] A 2018 study also found that oolong tea inhibits breast cancer growth.[27] **Herbal teas** are generally caffeine free and are made from a great variety of ingredients—everything from fruits to seeds (and sometimes not any tea leaves), though I wouldn't place any big bets on all those "slimming teas" that have cropped up in health food stores in recent years (and I certainly wouldn't recommend that you embark on one of those tea-only cleanses that has users chug gallons of milk thistle every day).

Other Drinks

I'd like you to eliminate all other beverages from your diet, at least for the first 15 days. As we move into the "rest of your life" phase, you'll be allowed some latitude in the occasional glass of red wine (or more at one of your biweekly free meals), but for now let's just stick with the basics of water and calorie-free drinks like coffee and tea. I'm not saying you can't ever have alcohol again—by no means—but its sky-high sugar content disqualifies it from the reset portion of our plan. So, for the next 15 days, just say no—then we'll talk about alcohol.

What Results Can You Expect to See?

According to the UN Food and Agriculture Organization, Americans have the highest daily consumption of calories in the world: more than 3,600 calories *per day*.[28] That's about twice as much as the U.S. Department of Agriculture advises an adult woman eats! Even more depressing is this: a 2015 report published in the journal *BMJ Open* revealed that Americans get more than half (nearly 58 percent) of their calories from junk foods like soft drinks, sweets, desserts, alcoholic beverages, and salty snacks.[29] No wonder we're so overweight!

The good news is that if you press the Reset button and change the way you eat for just these first five days, you will see immediate, and dramatic results. Just look at the chart that follows if you don't believe me!

Based on this chart, if your eating habits even vaguely resemble those of the "average American," you can expect to start dropping the pounds *immediately* on the Body Reset Diet. Instead of empty calories that stimulate your appetite without benefiting your body in any way, you'll be filling up with large amounts of protein and fiber designed to keep you feeling energetic and craving free all day and night. Even if you don't eat like the average American as in the chart, you may be consuming extra calories without realizing it. All you have to do is make the decision to lose the weight, and the pounds will come flying off.

	Average American Diet (calories)	Phase I Body Reset Diet (calories)
Breakfast	Bowl of cereal with 2% milk (400) and grande 2% latte (190) 590	White Smoothie (302)
Snack 1	Bottle of "pure" orange juice (240)	Veggies with almond butter (150)
Lunch	Bottle of soda (150) and foot-long BLT sub with mayo and cheese (720) 870	Red Smoothie (317)
Snack 2	Candy bar (320)	Low-fat popcorn (110)
Dinner	Chicken wings (400), mashed potatoes (250), and green beans (100) 750	Green Soup (220) and serving of lean protein (50) 270
Total Calories Consumed	2,770	1,149

What If You **Don't** Have a **Blender?**

We don't always have fresh produce and blenders available to us. But we can't use this as an excuse to fall off the wagon. When I'm in a jam, I like to use meal replacements (MRPs). These have all the essential components of the smoothie meals, including high-quality protein, fiber, healthy fat, and micronutrients. They come in two forms: powdered and liquid. The liquid form is conveniently available at most grocery stores and usually comes in a few flavors. Meal replacements also come in powdered form and can be made simply by adding water. I prefer powder most of the time because it's easier to keep on hand when I'm traveling. It fits in a desk, a purse, even a pocket. It's slightly more cost-effective, and you can customize it by adding additional ingredients if you want to add extra nutrients or flavors in the form of fruits, vegetables, or healthy fats. It has everything you need, tastes great, and is super convenient. A good meal replacement provides a similar nutrient profile to the smoothies and soups: 300–500 calories; 15–20 grams of protein; 10 grams of fiber; less than 10 grams of added sugar. The protein should come from a high-quality source, such as dairy (whey or casein) or egg white (albumin), and the fiber should not come primarily from a source that could upset your stomach, such as fructo-oligosaccharides, which are an indigestible form of carbohydrates that have been shown to have a potential to increase bloating, cramping, and symptoms of irritable bowel syndrome.

"I worked with Harley on *Revenge Body*. When I first learned about the details of the Body Reset Diet, I thought it was just too easy. *Why is he sending me home with a book, blender, an activity tracker, and telling me to just walk?* I wondered if it was too good to be true.

"The first two weeks, I dropped 14 pounds. By day 30, I had shed another 24 pounds. I could not believe it.

"I went from doing zero exercise to walking 10,000–14,000 steps a day and following a completely different diet. At the start, I had blisters on my feet from walking and hip pain, but after the first month of walking consistently, it became easier.

"My main motivation for being part of the *Revenge Body* process was to regain my self-confidence and self-worth. The mind–body connection is so strong, and negative self-talk can really be your biggest obstacle. Harley gave me the tools and support I needed to work on and overcome my issues and reignite my long-dimmed inner light.

"My advice to others: You can do it—no matter how busy you think you are. When I finally stopped making excuses, I started to see the results and changes in myself. This experience changed my life and I am forever grateful to the show, and more importantly, to Harley."

—CRYSTA, LOST 14 POUNDS IN 14 DAYS
(AND 24 POUNDS IN 30 DAYS)

7

Making the Smoothies

All right, now let's get down to the serious business of actually making the meals that you'll enjoy in the next 15 days. You'll have a white smoothie for breakfast, a red one for lunch, and a green soup for dinner, but you can interchange them as you please—as long as you're getting all three of them in each of the first five days.

The first rule I followed in coming up with these recipes is to be adaptable, above all else. I know everyone's tastes differ, so for all of my smoothies I offer slight and not-so-slight variations to suit a wide range of tastes, and to keep your palate entertained—after all, boredom has

Watch Your **Portions**

An important note: if you're a man or a woman who weighs more than 175 pounds, you need to increase the serving sizes by one-third to get all the nutrition and energy you need. In the three main smoothie recipes, I offer modifications in portion size to get you started. If you drop below 175 pounds over the course of this plan, then adjust your portion sizes accordingly.

been the death of many diets. It's important that you love what you're eating, so if apples aren't for you, toss in a pear or a peach instead. If you're not crazy about—or don't have—vanilla extract, use ground cinnamon.

To encourage improvisation, following each of the recipes for the basic White Smoothie, Red Smoothie, and Green Soup is a chart with suggestions for substitutions. Mix and match and see what pleases your taste buds. The important thing is that you find recipes that keep you coming back for more. By the time you're finished with this plan, you'll be an expert at building your own smoothies and soups with whatever you've got in the house.

STEP 1: MAKE YOUR SHOPPING LIST

Please, don't go to the grocery store on an empty stomach! And if you do, at least try to avoid the aisles with the most tempting foods if you don't think you'll be able to resist them.

The evening before you begin Phase I, buy all the ingredients you need to get through your first five days with ease. Remember, to avoid the pitfalls of yo-yo dieting, preparation is critical. I promise you, if you stick to this plan, you will NOT be hungry. Don't put yourself in a situation where you don't have the right ingredients for your lunch smoothie and so decide, just this once, to grab a quick cheeseburger instead. That's not going to fly, especially not during Phase I! Stock your pantry with the following foods so you'll have everything you need in advance to stay on track (and of course, look through the recipes and see if there are any that catch your eye that call for an ingredient not on this list before you go).

Phase I Shopping List

For smoothies:

> 5 red apples
>
> 5 small bananas
>
> 3 medium oranges
>
> 1 bag red or green grapes
>
> 5 pears
>
> 3 avocados (can use for soups, too)
>
> 1 bunch fresh spinach
>
> 3 limes
>
> 4 (10- or 12-ounce) bags frozen raspberries
>
> 2 (10- or 12-ounce) bags frozen blueberries
>
> 2 (16-ounce) bags frozen strawberries
>
> 1 (16-ounce) bag almonds (can also use for snacking)
>
> Ground cinnamon
>
> Almonds or 1 (16-ounce) bag almond meal, depending on the strength of your blender
>
> Plain or vanilla protein powder (see page 181 for a complete guide to buying protein powder)
>
> 1 (12-ounce) bag ground or whole flaxseeds or chia seeds, depending on the strength of your blender (Some, like the blenders I describe on page 31, will be able to grind the seeds themselves. Less powerful machines might require ground seeds.)

½ gallon fat-free, 1 percent, or 2 percent organic milk (or unsweetened nondairy milk of your preference)

1 quart fat-free, 1 percent, or 2 percent plain Greek yogurt (Chobani, Oikos, Fage, Trader Joe's, Siggi's, or Icelandic Skyr)

For soups:

1 head broccoli

2 medium zucchini

1 pound carrots (can be used for snacking, too)

1 box bouillon cubes (I prefer Knorr's)

Garlic powder

Onion powder

Don't Wait, Start **Today!**

Clients and readers often ask me what the best day is to start a diet, and I always have the same answer: today. The best time to start a diet is right now! But since you probably don't have some of the ingredients necessary to get you going, you might need to do some advance planning.

What's the beginning of your weekly cycle? For people who work Monday through Friday, I often recommend starting on a Saturday. You hit the grocery store Friday after work with your shopping list, then you wake up on Saturday and start blending. Over the weekend, you'll have more time to focus on perfecting your smoothies and adjusting to your new diet. By the time Monday rolls around, you'll already be on Day 3, or almost halfway through Phase I. You'll have momentum, and the confidence that comes with two days of smoothie making before the demands of the work week catch up with you. But like I said—any day is a good day, as long as it's soon. The important thing is getting started!

A **Rainbow** of Good Health

As with any food, there's a strong aesthetic component to the perfect smoothie, with those little stripes of orange and green and white all blended into a beautiful spiral. This pleasing appearance might stimulate your enjoyment of your drink, or so believe the Japanese, who think that a good meal should stimulate all five senses, including sight. The Japanese concept of *goshiki* states that every meal should have at least five colors: white (rice, tofu, or fish); yellow (scrambled eggs or squash); red or orange (carrots or sweet potatoes); green (any green vegetable you want!); and black, dark purple, or brown (eggplant or seaweed).

Goshiki ensures that a meal will please both the eyes *and* the palate—and in the process hit the main categories of ingredients that make up a well-balanced meal. We've pretty much lost this concept in North America, but I still believe that the aesthetics of a meal influence our enjoyment of it.

These colors have an important nutritional purpose, too. To bypass the boredom induced by most diets, which have you eat the same foods over and over, we've placed an emphasis not only on the macronutrients—the fiber, the healthy fats, and so on—but also on the micronutrients, and that's where the colors come in. Red foods are high in nutrients like cancer-fighting lycopene, while orange and yellow foods contain carotenoids, which boost the immune system and reduce heart disease risk. Blue foods are antioxidant powerhouses, and white foods, in addition to being a great source of potassium, might also reduce cancer risk. Green foods, of course, have endless benefits, as they contain everything from folates to lutein. So remember: colorful food doesn't just look good; it also has a direct impact on your health. To get the full range of nutrients you need, you should be consuming a whole rainbow of foods each and every day.

For snacks:

    1 pint fresh blackberries or raspberries

    1 small package high-fiber crackers, like Ryvita

    ½ pound low-fat cheese of your choice

    1 (5-or-so-ounce) bag air-popped, low-cal popcorn

    1 pound sliced turkey

    1 (12-ounce) package frozen or fresh peeled edamame

Snacks

When it comes to snacks, you're free to choose any protein- and fiber-rich snack that doesn't exceed 150 calories (for women) or 200 calories (for men). Make sure it has at least 5 grams protein, 5 grams fiber, and has no more than 5 grams fat or 10 grams of sugar. Refer to page 73 for a list of suggested snacks and choose several that you'll want to enjoy in the first five days. I'd pick up a pound of turkey, a package of edamame, some Ryvita crackers, a bag of baby carrots, and some hummus. Also, get some extra fruits and finger-food veggies just in case. Whatever you do, just make sure you have enough snacks for five whole days so that you don't go running to the vending machine.

STEP 2: SET A SCHEDULE

Starting today, you will be eating five times a day, every day, so to avoid getting too hungry, I want you to sit down and figure out in advance when exactly you'll be having your two smoothies, two snacks, and one soup. I want your first day on the plan to be a total success, so I really recommend you do this either the night before you begin or early in the morning of Day 1.

    Figure out times that work with your schedule, when you can realistically sit down and take 15 minutes for yourself. I like to eat at 7 a.m., 10 a.m., 1 p.m., 4:15 p.m., and 7:30 p.m. If it's easier to start on the weekend, when you have more control over your schedule, then by all means do that. Allow yourself the focus you need. The important thing is that you space these meals and snacks consistently so that you don't get too hungry and lose your resolve. Plan meal and snack times ahead so that your body will adapt to these intervals and know what to expect. It's all about conditioning from the inside on out.

For an example of a Phase I schedule, please see page 104.

STEP 3: MAKE THE SMOOTHIES

Now that you have everything you need on hand, it's time for your first meal!

Build Your Own Smoothies and Soups

And now for the ultimate mix and match of smoothie and soup making!

You can exercise a lot of creativity when it comes to making smoothies and blended soups—any and all fruits and vegetables are acceptable, as long as the overall profile of the meal fits our fiber and protein goals. So, pick an ingredient from each of the following categories and blend away!

You want to aim for a smoothie that has between 300 and 500 calories (the higher end of this range is if you weigh 175 pounds or more); 15 to 20 grams of protein; 10 grams of fiber; 15 to 20 grams of healthy fat; and less than 10 grams of added sugar (from your protein powder).

Ingredient Category

INGREDIENT CATEGORY #1: LIQUID BASE

Choose one

Water

Add as much as you prefer in your smoothies; and it's the best choice for your blended soups—especially the water you use to cook the vegetables in, as it will contain the vitamins and minerals that naturally leach out of your vegetables during the cooking process.

Milk, dairy

Fat-free, 1 percent, or 2 percent milk (¾ cup maximum)

Milk, nondairy (¾ cup maximum, and be sure to buy an unsweetened variety)

Almond milk

Hemp milk

Oat milk

Rice milk

Soy milk

INGREDIENT CATEGORY #2: PROTEIN

Choose one

Protein Powder

Whey protein

Casein

Egg white

Pea

Soy

Brown rice

Tofu (I like soft regular or silken tofu)

Yogurt

Fat-free or low-fat plain Greek yogurt

INGREDIENT CATEGORY #3: HEALTHY FAT
Choose one

Avocado

Nuts

Almonds

Cashews

Macadamia nuts

Walnuts

Peanuts (officially a legume, but we'll group it in nuts)

Seeds

Chia seeds (always add right before consuming so that they stay crunchy; otherwise they'll absorb your liquid ingredient and make your smoothie less drinkable and more of something you need to eat with a spoon)

Flaxseed

Pumpkin seeds, raw, unsalted

Sunflower seeds, raw, unsalted

INGREDIENT CATEGORY #4: HIGH-FIBER CARBOHYDRATE
Choose one

Fruits

While pretty much anything goes when it comes to fruits and vegetables, you should know that certain fruits have more fiber than others. Blackberries and raspberries, for example, are incredibly high in fiber, while bananas and melons are not. I'm by no means saying that you can't put bananas in your smoothies, but if you do, you also need an additional fiber source like chia seeds (which are also a healthy fat) or psyllium to meet the required nutritional profile. So, if you're making a piña colada smoothie, you need to make adjustments to compensate for the low fiber profile of both pineapples and bananas.

HIGHEST-FIBER FRUITS

Blackberries	1 cup	8 g
Raspberries	1 cup	8 g
Pear	1 medium, with skin	6 g
Orange	1 medium	4 g
Apple	1 medium, with skin	4 g
Blueberries	1 cup	4 g

Speaking of piña colada smoothies, certain fruits are also more calorically dense than others. You are absolutely permitted to eat them, but again, you'll have to make certain adjustments, principally when it comes to yield. Your piña colada smoothie will be somewhat smaller than your apple pie smoothie, since gram for gram, a banana is twice as calorically dense as an apple with only half the fiber. A smoothie built around raspberries or blackberries, on the other hand, is both high in fiber and low in sugar, so your serving size can be a bit larger.

HIGHEST-SUGAR FRUITS

Mango	1 cup	30 g
Red seedless grapes	1 cup	25 g
Papaya	1 cup	20 g
Banana	1 medium	20 g

LOWEST-SUGAR FRUITS

Cranberries	1 cup, raw	4 g
Raspberries	1 cup	5 g
Blueberries	1 cup	14 g
Grapefruit	1 cup	16 g

Vegetables

The sky's the limit when it comes to veggies, except when it comes to fat-based veggies like avocados and olives. I'm not saying they're bad—by no means—but for our purposes they belong with the healthy fats, not the high-fiber carbohydrates, and should be used sparingly.

The vegetables that blend best in smoothies are leafy greens. The champion of champions is spinach, which has a mild taste but still delivers all the amazing health benefits of these vegetables. As always, though, I recommend you walk before you run—that is, go for gentler spinach and lettuces before trying chard and kale.

As for the soups, a wide range of vegetables will work—that's why I included several options in the Master Green Soup recipe.

Leafy Greens
Spinach

Kale

Lettuce and salad greens (romaine, arugula, etc.)

Chard

Watercress

Other leafy greens (collards, mustard greens, bok choy, beet greens)

Good Veggies for Soups
Asparagus

Broccoli

Carrots

Cauliflower

Peas

Red bell pepper

Zucchini

Flavor Accents

Cinnamon

Ginger

Herbs (basil, mint)

Lemon

Lime

Vanilla

Bouillon (I like Knorr)

"I consider myself a pretty active person. I go to the gym at least three times a week and eat a pretty healthy diet. The problem is, I was struggling with the last 10–15 pounds. No matter how much cardio I did, I had definitely hit a plateau. Then I saw your book. I started the diet the next morning with the Apple Pie Smoothie. Wow! So simple and yummy! By the next morning I was running out of bed, had so much energy, and actually felt better.

"By the fifth day I was bouncing off walls, I looked leaner, and the belly fat I thought was a part of me since my cesarean section was almost gone. I told my husband this diet has become my new way of life. Ten pounds have come off so far and I am still seeing changes. I want to thank you again for this book, with its tasty and realistic recipes I feel like I have finally conquered the battle of the bulge."

—TANYA L., LOST 10 POUNDS IN 15 DAYS
(AND 18 POUNDS IN 6 MONTHS)

CHAPTER

8

Learning to Move

All right, now that you've got the eating part down, let's talk about exercise, yet another aspect of weight loss that has gotten completely out of control. Here, too, we desperately need to press the Reset button. Most people who want to lose weight fall into two categories. Some don't move enough, and others move too intensely. There's no greater symbol of this ridiculous extreme behavior than the fitness infomercials that flood our airwaves in the wee hours of the night. One popular fitness program is actually called INSANITY, which perfectly describes our state of mind, as well as the fitness fads we're so impulsively embracing one after the other.

Here's what these programs and the mind-set behind them are doing to us: We're getting injured. We have bad knees, bad posture, excessive soreness. And yet, we can't maintain a trim physique over the long term.

On the one hand, we're working out so hard, yet we're getting almost NO exercise in our day-to-day lives. How could we possibly take the stairs when our thighs are still aching from last week's SoulCycle workout?!

Spinning has gotten even more popular since the first edition of *The Body Reset Diet* appeared. And while anything that gets people excited about moving is a good thing, spinning tends to strengthen muscle groups that are already over-strengthened, including the quads and the calves, and doesn't do much for the typically underused muscle groups that are so important for good posture and injury prevention, including the glutes, and upper and lower back muscles. Also, the fact that your feet are fixed in place and your hips have to work so hard in only one plane of direction is a recipe for hip injury and even surgery—I have multiple clients who are facing these issues. Spinning should be just one tool in your toolbox—you can't undo six days of unhealthy living through 45 minutes of intense exercise

Our over-the-top exercise regimens are also supercharging our appetites and causing us to overeat, and overeating makes us fat. It doesn't help that when we work out so hard, we are blasting our bodies with huge amounts of the hormone cortisol, which studies have shown can increase levels of body fat.[1] Study after study has concluded that while moderate exercise has a protective effect on the body, improving general health and longevity, too much exercise can have the opposite effect.[2]

Stop feeling guilty about not going to the gym every morning before work. We have more gyms than any other country on earth—and more obese people. And why is that? Leaving aside our poor eating habits for the moment, one big reason is that we're not active enough in the right way. But wait, you say. Laziness is not my issue. I am a total gym addict. I go every single day after work. Fine, well—what do you do the rest of the time? The fundamental problem here isn't that we're not devoted enough to our burn-500-calories-in-an-hour spin regimen. It's that we've created this completely skewed situation in which we can exercise only at a certain time of day in a certain room in a certain building with a certain piece of equipment.

Our fitness hang-ups are yet another symptom of our efficient-to-a-fault lifestyles. Even if we do work out several times a week, we tend to spend the rest of the time not moving at all. Most of us sit at a desk for eight hours a day and spend another eight on the couch. Those of us who are exercising tend to be exercising too intensely and leading inactive lives, and the imbalance is catching up with us.

I have news for you: the manic exercisers who are so fond of going overboard at the gym are by no means at uniformly healthy body weights, nor are they particularly satisfied with their physiques. On the contrary, their weights tend to fluctuate regularly and in some cases dramatically for the reasons I've already described: they're injuring themselves, they're overeating, and because they're playing havoc with their stress hormones. Oh, and let's not forget that, like the rest of us, they're simply not moving enough in the rest of their lives.

These hard-core exercisers may well be investing time and sometimes serious money trying to get fit, but if they're eating an extra 1,000 calories a day for every hour they work out, they're ultimately undermining their efforts. To shed pounds, you *must* cut back on calories—but it's very hard to do this when you're running 12 miles before breakfast.

I'm not saying we don't need ANY exercise—not at all. Physical activity is extremely important, and our general lack of it is one of the main reasons we're so unhealthy as a culture. Activity improves our quality of life in ways big and small. It makes lifting suitcases and walking up the stairs easier; it relieves stress and improves posture. Regular movement boosts what the World Health Organization calls "healthy life expectancy," and it might even help us sleep.[3] It has a number of more surprising benefits, too, like boosting cognitive performance,[4] and helping to relieve mild to moderate depression.[5] A 2010 study showed that exercise can make cancer treatments more effective.[6] Exercise can help repair the body, as well as help to prevent injuries in the first place.[7]

So, yes, exercise is essential. But the big question is how much and what type.

First, we need to learn how to differentiate between "exercise" as we currently understand it—that is, something that can be done only inside a gym, at a designated time with a designated piece of equipment—and activity. Activity is a submaximal (below maximum) steady state of physical movement, a means of expending energy without forcing us to carve out a separate time from our days. Walking over to the copy machine, getting up to answer the phone, even fidgeting—all count as activity.

Unlike "exercise," physical activity is not scheduled or contrived but, rather, is a naturally occurring part of our everyday lives. And, most important, this type of regular, day-to-day movement does not cause our appetite to spike and induce us to eat more than we otherwise would. One 2018 study found that people who had just worked out were more subconsciously drawn to images of sweet treats immediately than those who either completed a puzzle or were given no intervention before viewing the images. The researchers theorized it could be an ingrained response aimed at quickly replenishing the calories burned during exercise.[8] The key, then, is not to sweat till you drop but, rather, to move constantly around the clock. Moreover, it's time to dispel one of the greatest myths around sweating: it doesn't equal burning fat! If you're sitting in a chair on a hot day and you sweat, you're not burning fat.

Instead of sending an email to your colleague ten cubicles away, walk over to ask the question in person. Instead of drinking your morning coffee in bed, throw on some sweatpants and drink it while strolling around the block. The list of possibilities goes on and on. Get up from your desk every 20 minutes. Buy a hands-free headset for your phone, and the next time you're on a call, take it while pacing your office or tidying the house. Don't just hunch over in your chair or stretch out on the couch. Leave your phone across the room so that you have to get up every time it beeps. Don't yell for someone else to answer the door when the UPS guy comes calling—get up and answer it yourself. When your favorite writer has a new book out, download an audio version of it and listen to it while walking to work instead of while lying in bed.

I promise you, all these little efforts will pay big dividends. Everything counts. Walking to the bathroom, going to the ATM on foot—all these movements contribute to your overall well-being. Even the smallest movements—what are known as incidental physical activities—can make a big difference in your overall cardiorespiratory fitness: a 2018 study found that replacing just a half-hour of being sedentary with everyday activity reduces risk of death from cardiovascular disease by 24 percent. This same study found that replacing sedentary behavior with just 10 minutes of brisk walking can reduce that risk of death due to cardiovascular disease by 38 percent—that's time well spent![9]

I guarantee that a person who's moderately active all day long—who always takes the stairs, who takes a lap around the office every 20 minutes—will be much healthier than someone who has a completely sedentary lifestyle but works out hard at a few pre-planned intervals several times a week.

This regular motion will have another side effect as well: it will keep you occupied, which is a good thing. Too often, overeating is a direct result of boredom and the desire for distraction, both of which are byproducts of our all-too-sedentary lives. So, whatever you do, get up and MOVE—especially while you're still getting the hang of this new system, when you're most likely to be tempted to snack for no reason.

How to Move in Phase I

I've said it before and I'll say it again: it's important to be physically active as long as you don't overdo it. It doesn't have to be vigorous or backbreaking. It just has to be regular physical activity.

That's why, for the duration of Phase I, we'll keep it super-simple on the exercise front, sticking to one and only one activity: walking. Walking is absolutely crucial to our continued good health, and it's a key determinant of countries with long life spans. One study found that women who walked at a moderate pace for as little as an hour a week significantly cut their risk of heart disease.[10] Regular walking has also been shown to reduce blood pressure, lower the risk of diabetes and strokes, and increase lung capacity.

A collaborative study involving fourteen researchers from the United States, Australia, Canada, France, and Sweden established preliminary guidelines for how many steps per day people should take for weight control, and the number they've hit upon is 10,000. The average adult American takes just 4,774 steps most days—is it any wonder we're so fat and unhealthy?[11] A 2019 study found that sedentary women, on average, took only 2,700 steps per day.[12]

So, 10,000 steps a day is the magic number here, a goal you'll be tracking with the help of an activity tracker, a step-counting device that you can easily keep in your pocket. Ten thousand steps is about 4 miles, which can sound like a pretty daunting number, but I promise you it's not; after all, we're counting every step you take from the minute you get up in the morning until the minute you go to bed.

For the first 15 days of this plan, you will carry your pedometer *everywhere* you go. You might be surprised by how much (or how little) you walk in an average day.

In the beginning, you might have to plot out exactly how to achieve this baseline goal of 10,000 steps. As with any life modification, there will be challenging moments, though I'd wager that these will be more psychological than physical. Getting to 10,000 steps can be as simple as taking a loop around the block before each meal or snack, or playing a game of pickup basketball for 20 minutes (which is how long it took me to hit 10,000 steps when I played last week). And whatever you do, make sure you take the stairs whenever possible.

Picking Out the **Perfect Activity Tracker**

Activity trackers—like a Fitbit, smart watch, or the classic pedometer—can have an impressive impact on how much you walk. Studies have shown that wearing an activity tracker can help increase people's awareness of their physical movements—and then, with any luck, increase their actual movements. A Stanford University study found that people who wore pedometers increased their physical activity by 27 percent, or about 2,000 steps (1 mile) every day. They also lowered their body mass index (BMI).

Activity trackers come at a range of prices; the most basic model can cost as little as $10 or you can get a base-model smart watch for around $400. They're also versatile devices. Some track your sleep, heart rate, and can let you answer texts, while others stick only to showing your step count. I am a big fan of the Fitbit because it tracks your number of steps accurately, as well as the intensity of those steps (in addition to tracking other biometrics such as sleep and heart rate), but if that isn't accessible to you, you can also investigate the many activity-tracking apps for your smartphone. Whether you want something simple and cheap or are willing to pay for bells and whistles, there's an option out there for you.

Easy Ways to **Hit 10,000**

- First thing in the morning, walk around the block.
- Leave the car at home and take the bus to work. Or, if public transportation isn't convenient, start a carpool with a neighbor and walk to that neighbor's house on foot.
- Get in the habit of parking in the most inconvenient, distant spot in the lot.
- Skip the escalator or elevator and take the stairs instead.
- At airports, skip the moving walkways and hoof it to the gate without technological assistance.
- Walk up and down every single aisle of the grocery store every single time you go shopping.
- Get a dog. Seriously, they have to be walked every day, regardless of weather, and that means they'll get you out walking, too.

I'm not saying that you can't *ever* use a treadmill at the gym—not at all. I'm saying that hitting the treadmill shouldn't be the be-all and end-all of your daily physical activity. Gym-going is a type of compensation for the exercise you're not getting in the rest of your life, meaning if it's 9 p.m. and you've managed to walk only 2,000 steps from the moment you woke up, then you need to either take a walk outside or spend a half hour on the treadmill. But these measures should be the exception, not the norm.

Remember, we are trying to avoid supercharging your appetite in these first few days. High-intensity bouts of exercise will not be assisting your efforts here. Instead, concentrate on reaching that 10,000-step mark before bedtime every night.

PHASE I SAMPLE SCHEDULE

6:30 a.m.	Wake up.
6:45 a.m.	After a shower, take your morning cup of coffee and walk around the block: 1,500 steps.
7:15 a.m.	Breakfast: White Smoothie
7:45 a.m.	Walk to the bus, or if you drive to work, make another quick loop around the block before getting into the car: 1,500 steps.
8:15 a.m.	Once at work, take the stairs, or arrive a little early so that you can take a quick walk to the newsstand a block away: 2,000 steps.
10:30 a.m.	Morning snack: 1 large Bosc pear + 2 slices of turkey. Walk downstairs and enjoy it on a bench outside: 1,000 steps.
1:00–1:15 p.m.	Lunch: Red Smoothie
1:15–2:00 p.m.	Spend the rest of your lunch break running errands on foot (picking up your dry cleaning, stopping by the coffee shop for another coffee). Or just catch up with your mom by telephone while you stroll through the neighborhood: 3,000 steps.
4:15 p.m.	Afternoon snack: 4 Finn Crisp crackers + 2 slices low-fat cheese. Now head down to a nearby coffee shop for an iced green tea to get you through those last few hours of work.
6:45 p.m.	Stop off at the grocery store on your way home. Remember to park in the most inconvenient spot in the lot, and be sure to walk every aisle: 1,500 steps. Congrats: you've hit your 10,000-step mark!
7:15 p.m.	Dinner: Green Soup

PHASE

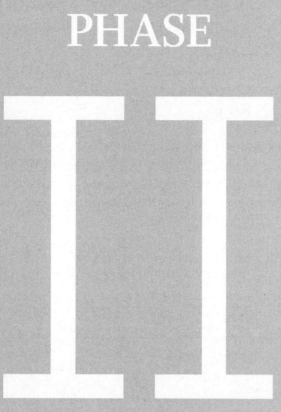

9

Making the Transition

Phase II: What You'll Be Doing

You will be eating five times a day: two smoothies (or one smoothie and one blended soup, depending on your preference), two snacks, and one single-dish meal. You will be upping your daily walking to a minimum of 12,000 steps and beginning a simple circuit of resistance training three days a week (or on Days 6, 8, and 10 of the plan).

What You'll Need

- A blender
- An activity monitor (e.g., Fitbit)
- A shopping list

You've done it! You've made it through the first, and surely the hardest, five days of the plan. I'd wager that you're looking and feeling pretty good right about now. How many pounds have you lost? Three? Five? Even more?

In any event, the dramatic results you've experienced in the last five days have surely been great motivation to continue on with the Body Reset Diet. I promise you it only gets easier at every phase as you gradually ease your way back into the "real world."

The biggest dietary change in Phase II is that you'll now be replacing one of your daily smoothies or blended soup with a satisfying single-dish meal (S-meal). I don't mind what time of day you eat your "real" meal—it really depends on your schedule and your eating habits.

Ask yourself when you're most vulnerable to pigging out and try to keep that meal as a smoothie or a blended soup. For me, dinner is the toughest time to stay disciplined, so that's the best time for me to have a smoothie or a blended soup. But efficiency is also a factor—when are you most crunched for time? If your morning routine is frenzied, maybe it makes the most sense to have a smoothie then, when you don't have time to prepare even the simplest meal. If it's quicker for you to bring your red smoothie to lunch in a thermos, then by all means do that, and have your S-meal at home with your family at night. If you like the ritual of slowing down and eating a meal with a plate and fork in the little park outside your office building, then bring your S-meal with you.

You can work out the details according to your own preferences and time constraints. There just has to be a method to the madness, so figure out what your method is.

Restoring a Passion for Eating

Sooner or later (preferably sooner), after a kick-start like Phase I of this plan, we have to make the transition back to single-dish meals. The smoothie is absolutely critical for the success of the kick-start: it is the most efficient, nutrient-packed way to shed pounds fast without devoting your entire day to obsessing about weight loss. But solid meals are better for long-term success, for a number of reasons. First, solid meals take longer to consume than even the most fiber-packed smoothies, and our bodies generally absorb them more slowly, both of which are good for weight loss. And there's a social aspect to eating that most diets overlook—and because they overlook it, those diets tend not to be sustainable. We are social creatures, and we can go only so long drinking every meal on our own.

There is also only so much variety you can get from a blender, and variety—of texture, flavor, and color—are important aspects of eating. Solid foods can give you a satisfying variety that smoothies cannot. Solid foods also take longer to digest, and sitting down to eat them is your chance to breathe and recharge. When you eat solid foods, your mouth acts as the blender, and you need to take time to ensure that it does its work properly.

Digestion, after all, starts in your mouth, both in its mechanical aspects, which set off a whole cascade of digestive processes in your stomach, and in the enzymes released by your saliva. When you slow down to chew every bite carefully, you'll increase the amount of nutrients absorbed into your body.

So, let's start to make the transition back to solid foods. Of course, whenever you get too busy or hectic, or feel the need to reset your habits again (or shed more weight in a hurry), you can always turn back to the three-blended-meals-a-day tool, but I don't really think it's realistic to live primarily off smoothies for the rest of your life. One smoothie a day, however, *is* sustainable, so that's what you'll transition to in Phase III and beyond.

Restoring a passion for eating is central to the long-term success of this plan. Yes, we all lead fast-paced lives and seldom come up for air. But when we pay too little attention to what we're putting into our mouths, we keep on eating and eating regardless of whether we're still hungry or even whether we like the food! I want you to reclaim not only a healthy lifestyle but also the enjoyment of the ritual of eating—gathering around the table with friends and loved ones, savoring every morsel of both food and conversation.

What You'll Be Learning: Basic Food Prep

The first thing I want to emphasize is that my recipes are EASY, so don't feel overwhelmed. The time commitment involved in making these meals will be 5 minutes or less, I promise. You *can* (and will!) prepare simple, delicious, and nourishing meals in a snap.

Taking control of your body (and what goes in it) does call for a measure of self-reliance in the kitchen, but that doesn't mean that cooking has to be a headache; on the contrary, these recipes will show you exactly how easy it can be to make great food.

Mastering Basic
Meal Preparation

Learning to prepare your own meals can fundamentally change the way you eat, and the Body Reset Diet meals are the perfect springboard for cooks of all experience levels, from gourmet chefs to total kitchen phobes. Studies show that people who prepare meals at home feel more emotionally rewarded after eating them. When you're preparing your own food, you also know exactly what's in every meal, which is not usually true of meals you order at restaurants or pick up in convenient little boxes in the freezer section of the supermarket. It should come as no surprise that food prepared at home tends to have a much lower calorie count than food ordered in a restaurant. An average restaurant meal contains between 1,000 and 2,000 calories, or between 50 percent and 100 percent of the total calories you should consume daily. By following the Body Reset Diet, you won't be frequenting restaurants as often as the average American, who eats out at least five meals weekly. Self-reliance in the kitchen and a tendency to eat more at home will yield big savings—in both the wallet and the waistline—over the years.

To show you just how simple cooking can be, we'll be starting with super-easy one-dish meals like stir-fries and soups that adhere to the basic principles of the Body Reset Diet, meaning they all contain a great balance of proteins, fiber, and healthy fats, and they all take under 5 minutes to prepare. Their nutritional profile—calorie count and fiber and protein content—is roughly equivalent to that of the smoothies; the main difference is that we consume them with a knife and fork instead of a straw or a spoon.

The key to these meals is SIMPLICITY, which is why I call them S-meals. The "S" stands for <u>S</u>imple, <u>S</u>ingle dish, and low <u>S</u>ugar, and also for the actual type of dishes:

- Salads
- Sandwiches
- Soups
- Stir-fries
- Scrambles

Simple = No Excuses. These meals are simple in terms of time, accessibility of ingredients, and preparation method—and simply delicious!

In Appendix D on page 217, I give you many options for each of these recipes. You can have Sweet Potato Hash with Chives (page 226) on Day 6, and try out the Southwestern Tuna Tortilla Wrap (page 239) on Day 7. To help keep things fresh, I've also added many new recipes, such as Kung Pao-ish Chicken (for when you've got a craving for takeout; page 274), a Shaved Sprouts Salad (when you want a delicious salad that you can take to work with you; page 258), and a 9-Minute Shrimp and Asparagus Stir-Fry (when you want a fancier meal that doesn't require a lot of time spent at the stove; page 272). There's something for everyone, and I promise that no matter how inexperienced you are in the kitchen, you *will* be able to make these meals in no time at all—and feel that much more satisfied with the food (and yourself) for having done it on your own.

Later, as you move into the Rest of Your Life phase, I encourage you to pick up some of my previous books to experiment with more delicious simple recipes, particularly *The Body Reset Diet Cookbook*. Those recipes are also incredibly filling, and a cinch to prepare no matter what your time constraints. But for now, let's stick to the one-dish meals, like the amazing Tuscan White Bean and Kale Bruschetta (page 278) and the mouthwatering Dijon Lentil Salad with Baby Spinach (page 265), which are truly as **<u>Simple</u>** as it gets!

Planning Ahead

Just as in Phase I, to succeed in Phase II you need to do some advance planning. Before you go to bed, think about what you'll eat the next day. Although this plan allows you to be flexible about what you eat, I do want you to continue alternating the smoothies in pretty much the same order, even as you go down to two a day. Over the years, I've found that establishing a routine helps you succeed in planning ahead to prepare meals. Obviously, the choices you make will really depend on your mood, and when you'll be in your kitchen and when you'll be on the move, and what you ate the day before and what you happen to have in your pantry.

The following chart is by no means a hard-and-fast template. It's merely an attempt to show you how you can alternate your meals and smoothies for maximum flexibility. If you strongly prefer the White to the Red Smoothie, then you can have the White Smoothie more often, but please don't exclude one type entirely. These smoothies were designed to give you the proper balance of nutrients when eaten in alternation. Try to rotate them.

The same goes for the S-meals. If it's the sweltering middle of summer, I totally understand that you won't be eating as many hot soups, but that doesn't mean you have to eat the exact same sandwich every single day. The success of a diet depends on variety, so try to eat as many different dishes as you can, especially early on when you're still figuring out what works for you.

PHASE II MENU GUIDE

	Day 6	Day 7	Day 8	Day 9	Day 10
Breakfast	White Smoothie (page 184)	Red Smoothie (page 186)	White Smoothie (page 184)	S-meal	Red Smoothie (page 186)
Snack 1	C-snack	C-snack	C-snack	C-snack	C-snack
Lunch	Red Smoothie (page 186)	S-meal	Green Soup (page 188)	White Smoothie (page 184)	S-meal
Snack 2	C-snack	C-snack	C-snack	C-snack	C-snack
Dinner	S-meal	Green Soup (page 188)	S-meal	Red Smoothie (page 186)	Green Soup (page 188)

Some Preliminary Tips for Transitioning Back to Solid Meals

- Try to eat your solid meals while sitting down (and no, driving doesn't count). Put down your phone, turn off the TV, and try to focus on what you're eating for the few minutes that you have. Enjoy your meals and you won't find yourself mindlessly snacking quite so often.

- Plot out your mealtimes well in advance. Don't get yourself in a situation where you're so ravenously hungry that you eat everything in sight.

- Chew your food slowly and deliberately.

- When you have eaten three-quarters of the food on your plate, wait several minutes and see if you're still hungry or if you can save that portion for leftovers.

"I found the Body Reset Diet from watching *Revenge Body* and within the first 7 days I lost 8 pounds, and after the full 15 days I lost a total of 16 pounds. I started at 276 pounds, which was my highest weight, and I am down to 260 pounds. It has forever changed how I see food and has provided me the foundation I needed to get started—and stay—on my weight loss journey."

—TAYLOR H., LOST 16 POUNDS IN 15 DAYS

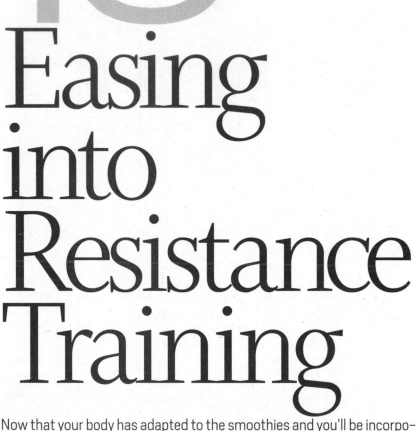

CHAPTER 10

Easing into Resistance Training

Now that your body has adapted to the smoothies and you'll be incorporating one solid S-meal into your daily diet, you're ready to up the number of steps you walk to 12,000 a day, and start a little resistance training. (Hitting 10,000 steps a day has gotten pretty easy already, hasn't it?) Adding resistance training and more steps are what take you from an active person to a fit person.

Resistance training—a type of strength training defined by resistance to a specific force of opposition—is an essential component of long-term good health. Resistance training can include everything from calisthenics (using your own body weight) to free weights. Pilates and yoga also fall into this category, though they are both submaximal forms of resistance training, meaning they have a good deal of value but aren't quite intense enough to create the visibly toned body we're trying to achieve.

According to the Centers for Disease Control (CDC), resistance training can be a powerful weapon against a wide range of maladies, from obesity and diabetes to back pain and arthritis. It has long been known that weight-bearing activity can improve muscle and bone density and therefore prevent osteoporosis.[1] Resistance training is our very best defense against chronic pain, and it can even fight depression. Additionally, it is particularly important as we get older, as it helps to counteract muscle atrophy and maintain mobility.[2]

While resistance training is not, strictly speaking, about burning calories—the point is more to sculpt your body and rev your resting metabolism to ensure that you're burning calories even when you sleep—its benefits are even more powerful for people trying to lose weight. Resistance training twice a week has been shown to improve resting metabolism and to reduce insulin resistance, body fat, and high blood pressure.[3] It's also the best way to tone and tighten your body; no diet, however healthy, can do this for you. But how much is enough?

As always, less is more. In spite of what you see at the gym or read in magazines, you do NOT have to go overboard. A 2012 study concluded that heavy weights aren't necessary for improving body strength: You can build the same amount of strength from lifting lighter weights more times as from killing yourself by lifting heavier weights a few times.[4] You don't have to push your muscles to their limit (and thereby

No Excuses!

The Body Reset resistance program could not be easier.
It doesn't require any equipment.
It takes less than 5 minutes from start to finish.
It consists of incredibly simple moves.

increase your risk of injury) to get the strongest body of your life. What matters more is being consistent and doing enough sets to tire out your muscles.

Together with your new diet, the Body Reset Diet circuits I've designed are THE shortest, simplest path to the strong, sexy body you've always wanted. The four exercises you'll do in Phase II are extremely easy to perform and take only 5 minutes out of your busy schedule, three days a week. *You don't even need any equipment*—no dumbbells or fancy gym machines—to see amazing results. (If you choose the more advanced exercises, you have the option of including a couple of dumbbells and a stability ball, but the program is otherwise equipment free.) The weight of your body is sufficient to get you in great shape in no time. Also, you don't need to do a million sets to start feeling serious and exciting changes in your body. Often doing one set can be just as effective as doing three or more, which is why we're starting you off with a single set.

Whatever your current fitness level, doing these circuits is a small investment with huge rewards.

Circuit A

In Phase II, you'll be doing Circuit A three days a week. This circuit consists of four simple exercises designed to train the *posterior muscles* of your body. These are the muscles attached to the back of your body.

The main posterior muscles we'll be working include:

- Your upper back (rhomboids)
- The back of your arms (triceps)
- Your lower back (spinal erectors)
- The back of your thighs (hamstrings and glutes)

Training posterior muscles is critical because over time our sedentary lifestyles have given rise to poor posture that can lead to major injuries. Every aspect of our daily lives causes us to hunch forward: we spend all day leaning into our computers, our phones, the steering wheel.

Our exercise habits aren't helping matters much, either. We do far too many crunches, chest flys, and biceps curls—exercises that work our already-overused anterior, or front, muscles. By doing more posterior than anterior work, we are undoing all the damage our lifestyles have done to our bodies over time. Not only do posterior muscles help correct our imbalances and address postural issues, but they can also make our arms and our midsections—the distance between our breastbone and belly button—look longer and leaner, giving us a natural chest lift. (This benefits both women *and* men—nobody wants flabby-looking pectorals!) Posterior exercises also drastically tone the back of your legs where your thighs meet your butt, and *everybody* wants that.

Depending on your fitness level going into the Body Reset Diet, you can modify the exercises as explained on the next few pages.

How Do I Know
If I'm a Beginner?

I've custom-designed these exercises for three different fitness levels: beginner, intermediate, and advanced. Here's how to figure out where you fall on the spectrum.

You're a *beginner* if, prior to starting the Body Reset Diet and getting your 10,000 steps a day, you were sedentary, you do not exercise regularly, and have done little or no resistance training in the past.

You're an *intermediate* if you've done some resistance training in the past and, before starting the Body Reset Diet, were somewhat active (i.e., you worked out at least twice a week).

You're an *advanced* if you're very familiar with resistance training and have been doing some form of resistance training two or three days a week (except perhaps during Phase I of the Body Reset Diet, when I counseled you to only focus on walking 10,000 steps a day).

How Many?

Beginners: Do 20 repetitions of each exercise; do one circuit.

Intermediate: Do 20 repetitions of each exercise; do two circuits.

Advanced: Do 20 repetitions of each exercise; do three circuits.

If you're starting as a beginner, you will add an extra circuit every month, until you are up to three circuits. When you have been doing three circuits for several months, you can progress to the intermediate and then the advanced movements. At the same time, you'll be adjusting the movements you're doing as your body gets stronger.

This progression—adding more repetitions and different variations as you acclimate to the exercises—is extremely important. For your body to progress, your fitness program must progress as well.

That's why I've built two different types of progression into this program: first, via the actual level of difficulty of the exercise (I offer modifications for beginner, intermediate, and advanced levels); and second, via the number of repetitions and sets of the exercise. You started in Phase I doing no resistance exercise—just walking—then proceeded to doing circuits three and then five times a week. As your strength builds, you will add more complicated variations and increase the number of sets you do. No matter which phase you're in, you'll always be walking at least 10,000 steps a day (12,000 steps a day in Phases II and III).

It's also important to understand that the key to resistance training is not the calories you'll burn while doing it but, rather, the residual increase in your metabolism that results from doing the exercises. The more toned our bodies, the more efficient our resting metabolism, and the more calories we burn—even while we're sleeping. In addition to walking 12,000 steps a day, you're continually burning fat *while* you're moving, but by doing these resistance exercises, you're training your body to burn fat *after* you're done moving.

How Often?

In Phase II, you will do Circuit A on three days: Days 6, 8, and 10 (and three non-consecutive days a week thereafter).

The Exercises

EXERCISE #1: REVERSE FLY

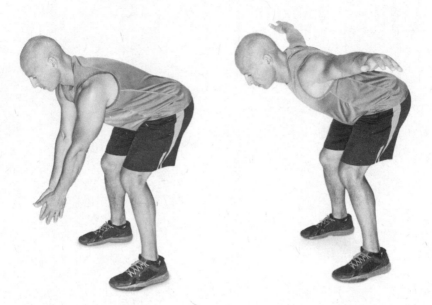

Works: Upper back and shoulders

How to: Stand with your feet shoulder-width apart. Stick your butt out and lean forward until your upper torso is parallel to the floor. Raise your hands out at your sides. (Imagine you are flying away—think of your arms as long wings.) Stop when your arms are parallel to the floor, then slowly lower your arms back down toward your sides. Keep a slight bend in your elbows throughout the exercise and squeeze your shoulder blades together at the top of the movement.

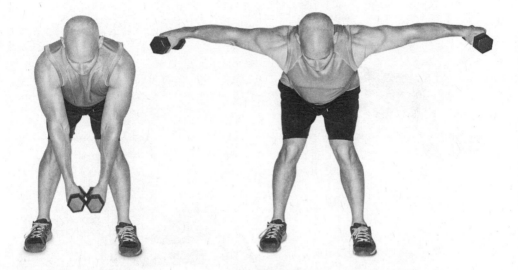

Intermediate: Add 16-ounce water bottles, one in each hand, first filled a quarter of the way with water, then halfway, then all the way, according to your strength level.

Advanced (*shown above*): Replace the water bottles with light dumbbells.

EXERCISE #2: TRICEPS DIP OR LYING TRICEPS EXTENSION

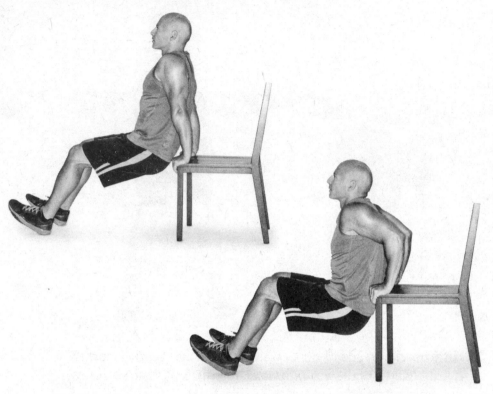

Works: Triceps primarily, but also shoulders and chest

How to: Begin seated on a bench or chair. Put the heels of your hands on the edge of the chair, slide your butt forward, and place your heels about hip-width apart on the floor. Slowly bending your elbows, lower your lower body 6 to 10 inches. Drive through the heels of your palm and contract your triceps. Now press your arms back up until they are straight. Repeat.

Intermediate: Extend your legs farther away from you. They can even be straight. The farther your feet are from your body, the more difficult the exercise.

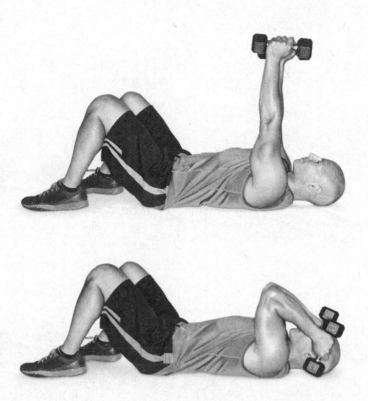

Advanced—Lying Triceps Extension (shown above): Lie on your back with your arms extended straight up toward the ceiling, your palms facing each other, and a dumbbell or water bottle in each hand. Hinging at your elbows, lower the weights down between your shoulders and ears, then extend them toward the ceiling and return to the starting position.

EXERCISE #3: SUPERMAN

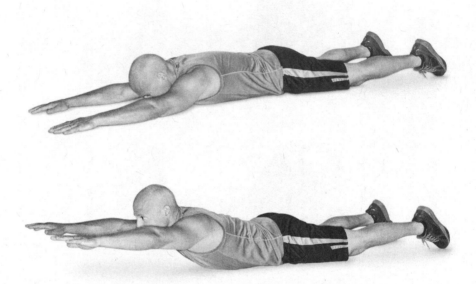

Works: Lower back and butt

How to: Lie facedown on the floor with your arms and legs fully extended. From this position, lift your arms toward the ceiling, as if you were flying. Lower back down and repeat.

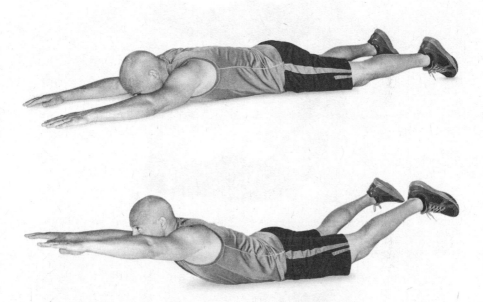

Intermediate: Add your lower body, lifting your legs at the same time as your arms so that your body looks like the letter X from above. Tap the floor with your hands and feet between reps.

Advanced: Don't let your feet or hands rest on the floor; keep them moving at all times.

EXERCISE #4: PRONE HAMSTRING CURL OR BALL HAMSTRING CURL

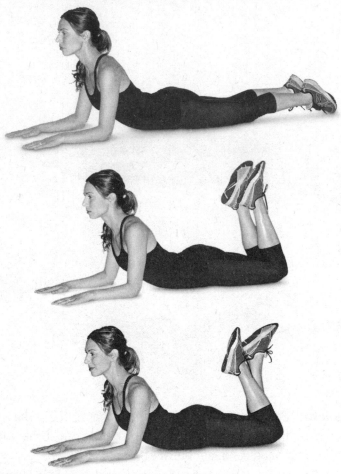

Works: Hamstrings

How to: Lie on your stomach, propped up on your forearms, with your hips down and your back as flat as possible. With your legs relaxed, bring your feet toward your butt.

Intermediate: Lie on your stomach, propped up on your forearms. Rest the laces of your right shoe on top of your left heel. (*See bottom photo.*) Repeat the exercise using your left hamstring, with your right leg working as dead weight. Do all the reps on your left leg, then repeat with your left shoe on top of your right heel.

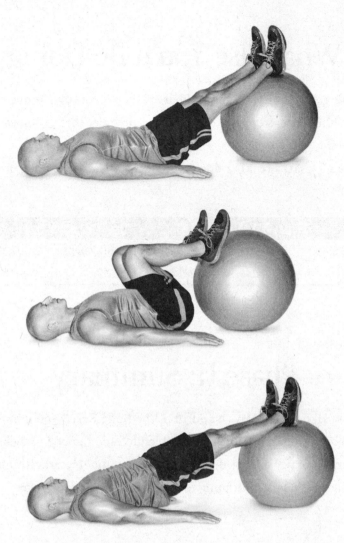

Advanced—Ball Hamstring Curl: If you're this advanced, you should invest in a stability ball. (You can buy one at any sporting goods store. The box will indicate, based on your height, which size you should use. Sizes vary from 45 to 85 centimeters; most people will probably use a 55–centimeter ball.) Lying on your back, put your heels up on the ball and lift your hips up off the floor. Keep your hips as high as you can manage. Bending at the knees, roll the ball in toward your butt and then back away from you.

What Else You'll Be Doing

Don't forget to keep walking! In Phase II, you'll continue to meet your goal of 12,000 steps every single day, so remember that pedometer and get moving.

Here's a chart breaking down your movements over the course of Phase II.

Day 6	Day 7	Day 8	Day 9	Day 10
12,000 steps	12,000 steps	12,000 steps	12,000 steps	12,000 steps
Circuit A	—	Circuit A	—	Circuit A

Phase II: Summary

In Phase II, between Days 6 and 10 of the Body Reset, you'll have two smoothies (or one smoothie and one blended soup), two C-snacks, and one S-meal a day. You'll be doing one short circuit of weight training on alternate days while continuing to walk 12,000 steps every day.

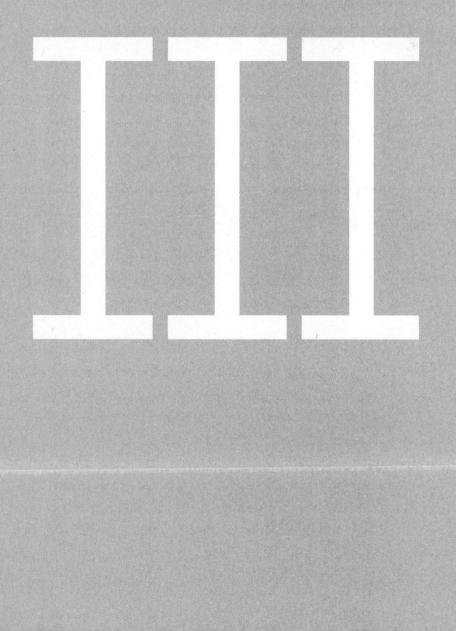

PHASE

III

11

Setting the Stage

Phase III: What You'll Be Doing

You will be eating five times a day: one smoothie or blended soup, two snacks, and two solid meals. You will continue to walk a minimum of 12,000 steps a day and add a second resistance circuit on alternate days. You'll still be doing resistance training just 5 minutes a day, but now you'll be doing it five days a week instead of just three.

What You'll Need
- A blender
- An activity tracker
- A shopping list

Phase III, which takes place between Days 11 and 15, is your launch pad to the rest of your life. The eating schedule that you will follow closely resembles—in slightly stricter form—the one you'll adopt once your 15-day reset is complete, meaning you will ultimately enjoy one smoothie or blended soup a day. You will continue to have two C-snacks daily, but you will also now have the option of two regular S-meals, choosing from the many great salad, sandwich, and scramble recipes I provide in this book.

Controlling Your Portion Sizes

As you prepare yourself to return to the "real world" of eating, you'll need to start thinking not only about WHAT you eat but also HOW MUCH you eat. You can eat the most nutritious ingredients in the world, but if you eat too many of them, you're still going to gain weight. It really is as simple as that.

If, on the other hand, you limit the size of your portions, you can eat pretty much whatever you want (within reason, of course). That's the primary reason the French, whose cuisine is among the richest in the world, are so much thinner than we are: they know that moderation is the key to success in eating.

A good deal of overeating is behavioral, related more to habit than to real need. One study found that children as young as 3 years old eat more food if more food is placed in front of them, and the same holds true as we get older: the more food we're served, the more food we eat. However, if we make an effort to limit our portion sizes, we will eat less food. A study found that people even feed their dogs more depending on the size of the bowl and scoop they use![1] The dogs fed with the largest scoops and bowls weighed more than those fed with regular-size scoops and bowls.

The same holds true for human behavior: It's no surprise that as the size of our dishware has increased in recent decades, so, too, has the size of our jeans.[2] In a 2006 experiment, participants were given either 34- or 17-ounce bowls and either 2- or 3-ounce serving spoons and told to serve themselves ice cream. The ones with the bigger bowls took 31 percent more ice cream, and the ones with the bigger spoons took 14.5 percent more. Those given both the larger bowls *and* the larger spoons took a whopping 56.8 percent more.[3]

Start paying closer attention to serving sizes, and be mindful of everything you put in your mouth. Though obviously superior to almost any food out there, even certain good-for-you fruits can cause weight gain if eaten in massive enough quantities.[4] Always pay attention to quantity, and know when to say when.

Here are some great tips you can use to control portions:

- Fill up on green salads and soup before the main course. (But avoid full-fat dressings and bacon bits!)

- Choose smaller plates so that your eyes don't trick you into eating more food than you need. A reasonable portion of food will be dwarfed by a gigantic dinner plate, so consider eating off smaller side plates.

- Pack your snacks in advance to limit how many you eat. If you have a single-serving bag of soy nuts with you, you will eat only that small bag. If, however, you bring a large package, you are *much more likely* to go overboard and exceed the ½-cup portion.

- Don't eat in front of the TV or computer—there is no better way to lose track of what you're eating (and therefore to eat much more of it than you need) than to eat when you're not paying attention.

- Don't eat buffet-style (except when it comes to salads and fruits). Remember—the more food that's in front of you, the more you're likely to eat. It's easier to avoid having seconds if you have to cross the room to refill your plate.

- Stick to the eating schedule you've used in Phase I and Phase II, and make sure you are eating five times a day, and that each snack and meal has plenty of fiber and protein to keep you full and prevent that "hangry" feeling that causes you to gorge on whatever you can get your hands on.

Planning Ahead

As you continue the transition away from the reset part of the Body Reset Diet, it's more important than ever to figure out when exactly you're going to eat. Is it simplest for you to have your daily smoothie first thing in the morning, when you're trying to do ten things at once before rushing out the door to work? Then by all means do that. Is it too much trouble to pack a sandwich to take to work and easier to have eggs at home and pack a smoothie to go? Then try that instead.

Again, as long as you plan your mealtimes in advance and try to get as wide a variety of Body Reset Diet foods into your days as possible, you can alternate the foods according to your taste and your schedule. The following chart shows you how easy it is to organize your meals in Phase III.

PHASE III MENU GUIDE

	Day 11	Day 12	Day 13	Day 14	Day 15
Breakfast	White Smoothie (page 184)	Italian Flag Breakfast Pizza (page 220)	White Smoothie (page 184)	Onion, Turkey Sausage, and Spinach Frittata (page 218)	Red Smoothie (page 186)
Snack 1	C-snack	C-snack	C-snack	C-snack	C-snack
Lunch	Coconut Chicken Curry (page 279)	Red Smoothie (page 186)	Southwestern Tuna Tortilla Wrap (page 239)	Easy Niçoise Salad (page 268)	Tzatziki Chicken Flatbread (page 241)
Snack 2	C-snack	C-snack	C-snack	C-snack	C-snack
Dinner	9-Minute Shrimp and Asparagus Stir-Fry (page 272)	Sweet Potato Hash with Chives (page 226)	Black Bean Soup with Lime (page 250)	Green Soup (page 188)	Grilled Steak and Baby Spinach Salad (page 264)

"My husband and I moved out to the burbs to be close to my new job. We bought a car and no longer walk everywhere, and we gained quite a bit of weight in just a few months. Despite trying to eat healthy, we were not able to shed the pounds.

"We just finished our 15-day program and we've both lost over 9 pounds each! More than that is the fact that I feel 10 years younger: I sleep better, wake up refreshed, and have more energy during the day. Your recipes are fantastic! (Our favorite is the Coconut Chicken Curry.) This started as a diet but it has become a lifestyle. It has simplified the processes of grocery shopping and food preparation, and has significantly reduced the grocery bill."

—JIM & MICK Z., EACH LOST 9 POUNDS IN 15 DAYS
(AND LOST 34 POUNDS AND 31 POUNDS, RESPECTIVELY, IN 6 MONTHS)

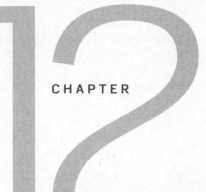

CHAPTER

12

Increasing the Resistance

The resistance–training component of Phase III is just an extended version of the easy, at-home exercises you've gotten in the swing of doing during Days 6 through 10. It still takes only 5 minutes a day, only this time you'll be alternating between two sets of exercises five days a week.

The Phase III program consists of Circuit A, which you mastered in Phase II, to work all the posterior muscles of your body, and Circuit B, which works all the anterior muscles, or the muscles at the front of your body.

The main anterior muscles we'll be working include:

- Your chest (pectorals)

- Your sides (obliques)

- The front of your thighs (quads)

- The front of your midsection (rectus abs)

You'll do Circuit A (descriptions and demonstrations of exercises start on page 146) on Days 11, 13, and 15; and Circuit B on Days 12 and 14.

Notice how you end up doing three Circuit A routines and only two Circuit B routines per week? That's no accident: It's our way of correcting the muscle imbalances that have built up in our bodies over time. By consistently favoring the anterior over the posterior muscles, we are giving the underused muscles on the backs of our bodies a chance to catch up with our overburdened fronts. That's also why we're doing a plank instead of a crunch, which strengthens the front of our bodies without putting strain on our backs. It's important to work both the anterior and posterior muscles to maintain a straight, strong posture. It's not only good for our bodies but it helps us look great in our clothes, too!

Circuit B

Again, in Phase III, you'll be doing Circuit A three times and Circuit B twice. Depending on your fitness level going into the Body Reset Diet, you can again modify the exercises as described.

How Many?

Beginners: Do 20 repetitions of each exercise; do one circuit.

Intermediate: Do 20 repetitions of each exercise; do two circuits.

Advanced: Do 20 repetitions of each exercise; do three circuits.

How Often?

In Phase III, you will do Circuit A three times—on Days 11, 13, and 15—and Circuit B twice—on Days 12 and 14.

"Originally, I was going to do the Body Reset Diet by myself, but as I was reading the first few chapters of the book, I knew this was something that could work for both me and my husband. Jason was skeptical at first, but the more I told him about it the more he was on board. He started the plan at 499.8 pounds and has lost 14. I started at 276 pounds and have lost 7.

"We have obviously tried other plans and they just didn't work for us. We have both been having some health problems, high blood pressure for example, and knew we had to make a change. Both of us are 32 and are too young to be having health issues like this. Finding *The Body Reset Diet* when we did was perfect timing. We were ready for a change, a major one, but it had to be healthy and something that would teach us how to eat and maintain a healthy lifestyle.

"Staying on plan has helped our wallet, too! No restaurant food for 15 days is saving us money and showing us how easy it can be to eat at home. While my husband is excellent in the kitchen, I am not, so having easy-to-prepare meals really helps me out!"

—NAHTANHA K. AND JASON K., LOST 7 POUNDS AND 14 POUNDS, RESPECTIVELY, IN 10 DAYS

The Exercises

EXERCISE #1: SQUAT OR SKATER LUNGE

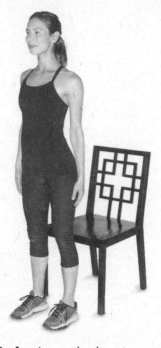

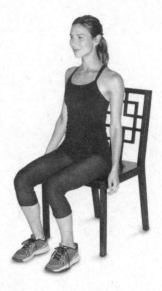

Works: Lower body (glutes, quads, hamstrings)

How to: As you squat and lunge, keep your weight on the arches of your feet and try not to roll onto your toes. Keep looking up the whole time and never lower your butt past your knees. Your thighs should end parallel to the floor.

Intermediate (*shown at right*): Use a lower seat and continue to sit onto it as before. If you'd like to make it even more difficult, hug a watermelon or add a set of light dumbbells.

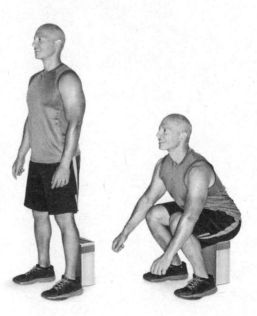

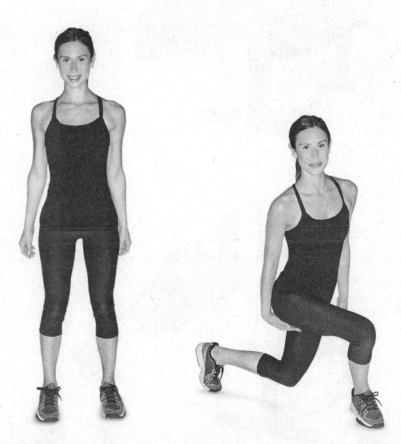

Advanced: Now you're ready for the Skater Lunge. Stand with your feet shoulder-width apart. With your right leg, step back and across your body, dropping your right knee behind your left heel. Then return to the beginning stance and do the opposite—step your left leg back and across your body, dropping your left knee behind your right heel (as shown above). Keep alternating legs, bending one knee to the opposite heel.

EXERCISE #2: MODIFIED PUSH-UP

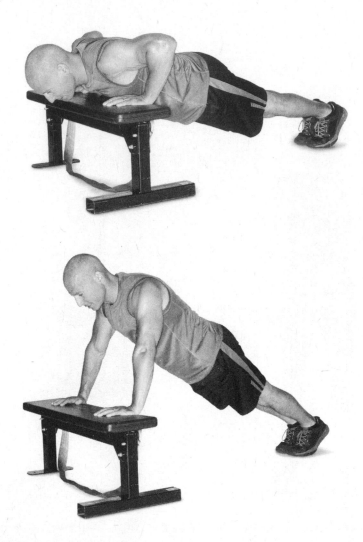

Works: Chest, shoulders, triceps

How to: Lean against a bench or countertop. Keep your body rigid and in a straight line. Line up your hands right above your collarbone and nipple line. Bend your elbows and slowly lower your body toward whatever surface you're using. Extend your elbows and repeat.

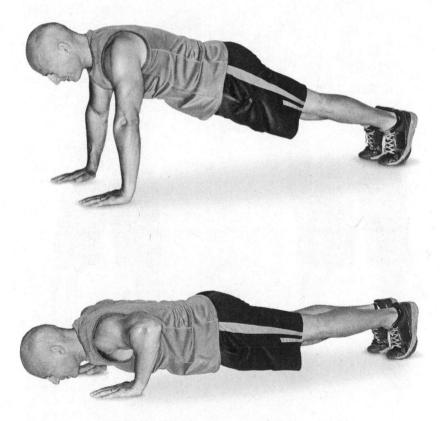

Intermediate: Perform this exercise on the floor with your knees bent and touching the floor and your ankles crossed behind you.

Advanced (*shown above*): Do a full push-up, with your knees off the floor and your entire body raised.

EXERCISE #3: STANDING SIDE BEND

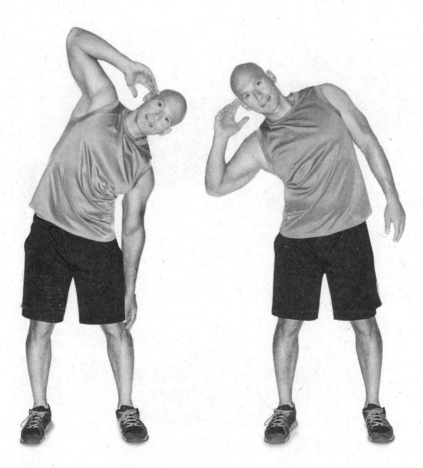

Works: External and internal obliques (aka "love handles")

How to: Stand with your feet shoulder–width apart, with your right index finger and middle finger behind your right ear and your left arm straight against your side. Gently lean your upper body to the right. Repeat in the opposite direction.

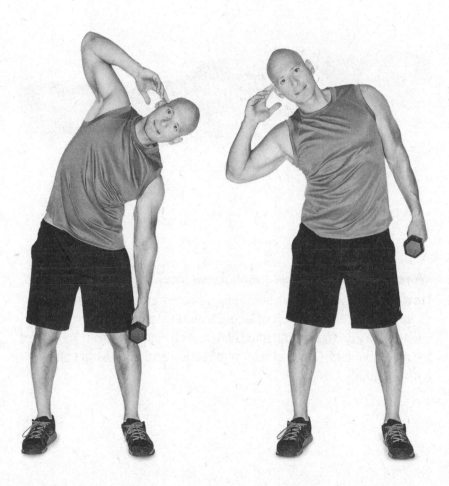

Intermediate/Advanced: Do the exercise with weights—a grocery bag full of canned food, a jug of water, or a dumbbell—in your straight arm.

EXERCISE #4: PLANK

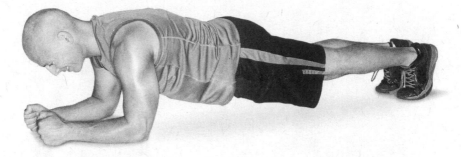

Works: Rectus abdominals (front of your core)

How to: With your elbows bent, rest your forearms on the edge of your bed, or the arm rest of a couch, and extend your legs back so your feet are on the ground and there is a straight line from your heels to your shoulders. Contract your midsection and form a rigid plank with your body.

Intermediate (*shown at left*): Now perform the same exercise on the floor. Rest your forearms on the floor but allow your hips to be slightly above the plane of your body.

Advanced: Perform the same exercise but make sure your hips are in a straight line with your shoulders and heels.

What Else You'll Be Doing

Meeting your goal of 12,000 daily steps should be second nature by now, allowing you to focus on the expanded resistance training.

The following is a chart to break down your movements over the course of Phase III.

Day 11	Day 12	Day 13	Day 14	Day 15
12,000 steps	12,000 steps	12,000 steps	12,000 steps	12,000 steps
Circuit A	Circuit B	Circuit A	Circuit B	Circuit A

Phase III: Summary

In Phase III, between Days 11 and 15 of the Body Reset Diet, you'll have one smoothie, two C-snacks, and two S-meals a day. You'll be alternating Circuits A and B of resistance training while continuing to walk 12,000 steps every day.

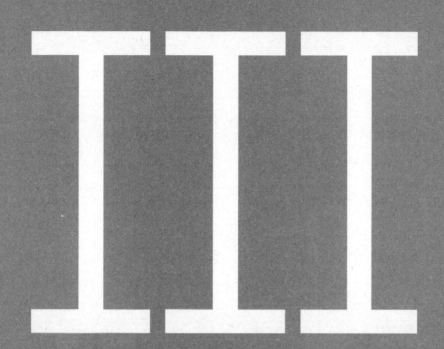

III

The Rest of Your Life

CHAPTER

13

You
Then
and Now

You did it! You made it through the 15-day reset, and you're probably feeling (and looking) pretty amazing right about now. You're finally ready to start incorporating your healthy new habits into your life for the long haul, embracing a lifestyle change that you can sustain for years to come.

First, let's check your progress. Just look at all you've achieved already! In just 15 days, you've lost weight, toned up your body, reset your palate to enjoy the taste of whole foods, weaned yourself off added sugar, trained yourself to eat five times a day so that you ward off cravings, and saved money without sacrificing any time from your already-packed schedule.

Here's how it works going forward. Like I keep saying, so many diets fail because they don't take into account how the real world actually works: how busy we are, how stretched our budgets are, how easily discouraged we can become. Once you get to the end of Day 15, you can—and will—keep going. Just continue doing what you've already been doing! The only difference is that now you're able to enjoy two "free" meals a week during which you can eat and drink whatever you want!

That's right, two meals of your choice. Why? Because life isn't about deprivation. It should be enjoyed and it's okay to occasionally eat your favorite foods, as long as you're following this plan for your other meals the rest of the week.

Getting Creative

As you get more confident with your blender (and you'll see that it doesn't take long at all), you can also follow the Build Your Own Smoothies and Soups guidelines I lay out starting on page 89, which couldn't be more straightforward: as long as you hit all the major nutritional categories—fiber, protein, healthy fat—you can experiment to your heart's content. Just don't forget that a smoothie without one of these key categories doesn't count as a meal, so if you throw bananas, strawberries, and ice cubes into a blender, you're not getting the protein you need to stay full until the next meal.

Hitting **Reset** Again

Whenever you need to lose a few pounds fast—say, after the holidays or a particularly indulgent long weekend—you can easily reintegrate Phase I or II of the Body Reset Diet, either for one day or for the full five days, or any number in between. Even a temporary reset can serve as a great detox at a moment's notice, without forgoing any essential nutrients. Reverting to Phase I in particular can help you lose weight in a hurry if you have a big event coming up and want to tighten up a bit, or just feel like you need an extra boost.

But the timing is entirely up to you. It really just depends on what type of reset you want and what your body needs at the time. Maybe you will revise Phase II for a little tweak once a month, or Phase I once a season, just to turn over a new leaf. That's what I like to do: drink three blended meals a day for the first five days of summer, fall, and so forth, for a fresh start. However you choose to use it, this plan is always there for you when you need it!

When you choose to have your daily smoothie or blended soup is still entirely up to you. I'm always doing ten things at once from the second I get out of bed, so I generally opt to have a smoothie for breakfast, cycling through the red and white smoothies (I *love* the PB&J Smoothie; page 200) depending on my mood and what I happen to have in my fridge. The rest of the day I eat as I always have: two meals and two snacks that all contain a healthy blend of fiber, protein, and healthy fat. You can also choose to have your daily smoothie or blended soup at the time of day that you might be most vulnerable to bingeing.

The one big (and I'm sure welcome) change in this phase is that you'll now get to have two "free" meals a week—that is, meals when none of the rules apply.

Bonus Perk: The Free Meals

As your reward for making it through all 15 days (as if your looser-fitting jeans weren't enough), you can now incorporate two weekly "free" meals into your diet. At free meals, you can eat and drink whatever you want. You can enjoy these meals as a Sunday brunch, a Friday night dinner with friends, or a date night with your significant other. It's completely up to you.

Why these "free" meals instead of the "cheat day" I included as part of my 5-Factor plan in a previous book? Well, many popular diets (including mine) have a cheat day, but I've found that just calling it by that name makes people feel compelled to not just indulge but also to over-indulge, and even to abuse their bodies. I've had clients who'd even wake up extra early on their cheat day so they could have more hours to jam down pancakes and hamburgers and pizza. Nope, I am not making this up. (P.S.: Thank you to all my Facebook and Twitter friends—I polled you all and you pretty much unanimously chose two free meals over one cheat day!)

So after much consideration, I've gotten rid of the word "cheat" because you're not really cheating anything; you're just ignoring the structure governing the rest of the week. "Free" can have a multitude of meanings. Maybe it means that you eat a healthy meal but have dessert, or maybe it means that you have a few drinks with your meal—"free" can mean whatever you want it to mean.

Another advantage of the two free meals over the one cheat day is that dedicating a whole day to cheating meant people felt they had to be completely perfect for the other six days, and that's really difficult. Often, people have a social event (or two) during the week, and I don't want anyone to quit the whole program because it doesn't accommodate his or her social life. Getting two free meals a week is better for your social life—and your body. After all, a cheat day means up to three meals and two snacks of cheating, whereas two free meals a week is exactly that—two meals—so it's less than half as much indulging.

This plan is all about lasting years, not days, and I find that too much deprivation and too-stringent regulations can often produce an unwanted backlash. You feel resentful when you are always denying yourself the treats you used to love, so instead

Alcohol: **A Few Cautions**

Alcohol has nearly twice the calories of carbohydrates and protein per gram, but that's not my main concern with it. I'm more worried about the enzymatic environment created by the consumption of alcohol. When we consume alcohol, our liver has to work over time to create the enzymes necessary to metabolize it. But our liver is also responsible for metabolizing fat, so when it's working on metabolizing the alcohol, it's not creating the enzymes necessary to burn fat. So, put simply, *when we drink alcohol, our bodies are doing a less efficient job of metabolizing fat.*

More obvious, perhaps, and equally pernicious are the behavioral hazards of drinking alcohol. When we're under the influence of booze, we have a tendency to eat with abandon. I consider alcohol a gateway drug of sorts—not necessarily for more drugs but for poor food choices. That said, as I learned when researching *The 5-Factor World Diet,* many of the world's healthiest countries include alcohol as part of their lifestyles, though always in moderation. If you exercise caution and indulge only at your free meals, you can enjoy alcohol without endangering your newly slim waist. So, it's fine if alcohol is your splurge, but let it be part of your free meals.

of sticking to the straight and narrow, you find yourself bingeing more and more. That's why I really prefer you treat these free meals as special occasions—rewards for how great you are doing— rather than just eating an entire box of sugary cereal in front of the television.

Never feel guilty about what you eat at your free meals; after all, you've earned them. Eating badly twice a week is still much healthier than eating sort of badly around the clock. It's the accumulation of carbohydrates and sugars day in and day out that does your body the most harm, not the rare indulgence. So, go on out and have fun! And look at it this way: if you're eating 35 times a week (21 meals and 14 snacks) and splurging on just 2 of those, then you are still way ahead of the game.

I've also found that, if you take these free meals in the context of an otherwise healthy diet, you might not find those old junk foods quite as tempting as you once did. You might experience a sugar headache, or indigestion, from the assault of processed foods on your newly pristine body. You'll be less tempted to eat and drink to excess; your body just won't want the same poisons anymore.

So go on and head out to your favorite Mexican restaurant and dig into that chip basket. Have a slice of carrot cake, if you so desire; it's your free meal, so there are no limits. You can even have alcohol, though I've offered a few general health reservations about it (see previous page).

Of course, the bottom line here is that life is meant to be lived, and I'm not going to tell you *anything* you cannot do on your two free meals a week. That's why they're free! You can eat or drink absolutely anything you want, though if you want to keep your alcoholic beverages on the healthier side, I'd suggest avoiding sugary drinks like piña coladas and daiquiris. But regardless; it's YOUR free meal, so go ahead and indulge to your heart's content. Like I said, you've earned it.

> "My sister and I don't think the diets in the past worked for us because we weren't ready and they were just fads. Reading Harley's book and being on his program made us realize that it wasn't a diet at all—it was a lifestyle change. Eating five small meals a day with the protein and fiber we needed was a great combination with our workouts. Our families were—and still are—amazed by our weight loss. We will tell anyone: it starts in YOUR mind."
>
> —JAMILLA AND CHERRELL H., *EACH LOST 9 POUNDS IN 15 DAYS*

Tips for Long-Term Eating Success

Plan, plan, and plan some more. I know I'm getting a little repetitive on this subject, but one of the most effective ways to ensure your continued success on this plan is to plot out your mealtimes well ahead of time. Don't leave anything to chance and get into a situation where your blood sugar is so low and your hunger so raging that you will eat everything in sight and then some. If you plan your meals and snacks at intervals of about 3 hours, you are far, far less likely to fall into this trap. But obviously, every day (and every mood) is different, and if you do feel hungry unexpectedly off your usual schedule, reach for a calorie-free beverage to see if that helps alleviate the pangs. And if planning works for you, consider also keeping a food journal, which has been shown to promote weight loss.[1]

Be mindful of why you're eating. Often, we don't eat because we're hungry. We eat because we're stressed or bored or unhappy. The best cure for this vague discontent is activity. If you're spending four hours a night watching TV on the couch, you're going to snack more. But if you're spending those same hours gardening in the backyard or playing tennis with an old friend, then by default you won't be snacking mindlessly quite so often.

Cover all your bases. Remember, to give your body the fuel it needs to thrive—rather than filling it with a bunch of empty calories that drag you down—you want to hit a few basic categories at every meal or snack. You've got to have fiber, and you've got to have protein. Without those two elements, your body is going to crave more food sooner than it needs it. Whenever you buy packaged foods, check the label to make sure they contain at least 5 grams of fiber and protein and weigh in at under 150 calories per serving.

Slow down—and stop while you're ahead. Get out of the habit of gorging yourself every time you sit down to eat. Chew thoroughly before swallowing, and make an effort to leave a few bites on your plate, just to see if you can. And take a cue from the Japanese, who try to stop eating when they're 80 percent (instead of our habitual 200 percent) full. Instead of lunging for the dessert tray right away, Japanese are raised to wait 5 to 10 minutes to see if they still want food. The vast majority of the time, they don't—and you won't, either. Try it on your next free meal. You might be impressed by your own self-control!

> "My best advice to anyone starting on a journey toward health and wellness is to start right now. Not tomorrow, not Monday, but NOW. Make the commitment and stick to it. This isn't a diet—it's a lifestyle change! While it can be challenging, what better

reward is there than a life of health, wellness, and feeling good about your body?"

—DELIA L., LOST 11 POUNDS IN 15 DAYS

Stock up on healthy foods in advance. Knowing what not to buy is one thing, but knowing what TO buy is just as important. I find it helpful to keep my pantry and fridge stocked at all times with healthy staples that I can turn into delicious meals in seconds flat.

- For smoothies: I go through stretches when I stock up on large quantities of spinach, frozen berries, fat-free Greek yogurt, and almonds—all of which I buy in bulk.

- For stir-fries: I always keep a bag of sliced veggies in my freezer in case of emergency.

- For scrambles: I buy a big carton of egg whites.

- For sandwiches: I buy whole grain, high-fiber bread (at least 5 grams of fiber per serving) and I freeze it, making it last longer.

- For salads: I go with fresh veggies, buying whatever's in season or on sale at my local market.

- For soups: I sometimes double or even triple the recipe so that I can freeze extra portions for when I'm in a hurry but want to eat something on the plan. This is an especially helpful tip during the winter months. I also buy low-sodium chicken or vegetable bouillon and fibrous vegetables like cauliflower and broccoli to throw in the blender.

Clean house. If you want to stick to this plan, it's a good idea to get rid of all the high-sugar foods in your house. You don't need to be tempted by sweetened cereals and fattening cookies in your life, so why do you have them in your kitchen? Replace anything with the words "hydrogenated" or "high fructose" with delicious whole foods so that you won't fall prey to temptation in weak moments. (We all have them.) Many of the toughest battles take place in the snack-food aisles of the grocery store, so show up with a list and stick to your goals. Having kids is no excuse: they don't need those unhealthy foods, either. Nuts, fruits, and low-fat cheese sticks make a much healthier after-school snack than the usual junk we give our children. If other people in the house insist on keeping junk food around, keep it in a specially designated cupboard, not at eye level.

Order wisely. Yes, you *can* eat whatever you want at your free meals, but try not to leave all your hard-won knowledge about health and nutrition at the restaurant door. In particular, remember that a meal isn't a meal without protein and fiber, so try to keep that in mind when you're scanning the menu of your favorite restaurant. Also, as always, pay attention to portion sizes, which tend to be gigantic everywhere we go these days. Avoid the bread or chip basket if you can—that's one of the big reasons we eat so much (often without even noticing) when we go to restaurants. If you save your appetite for the main event, you might find that you enjoy the food more. Getting in the habit of taking a doggie bag home with you is a great way to save on calories without restricting your favorite foods. Ask for it when you're ordering to limit temptation. Instead of wiping your plate clean, try to save a portion of your meal for lunch the next day, or bring some home for a (sure to be grateful) family member. Don't be afraid to ask for dressing and sauces on the side.

Stick to a schedule. Yep, keeping a consistent schedule is important, if not more so, in this lifelong phase. Get into the habit of knowing what you're going to eat beforehand. At the beginning of the week, try to have some idea of when you'll be taking your free meals. Make sure your kitchen is stocked with the foods you need to make a smoothie every day and healthy S-meals and C-snacks the rest of the time. Before going to bed at night, have an idea of what you'll be eating when you wake up. The same advance planning that got you through the first 15 days with such ease will be an invaluable resource as you adapt this way of eating to the rest of your life. The following chart will guide you through the first five days of planning how you'll be eating for many years to come. It should be old hat by this stage!

EATING PLAN FOR THE REST OF YOUR LIFE

	Monday	Tuesday	Wednesday	Thursday	Friday
Breakfast	White Smoothie (page 184)	Italian Flag Breakfast Pizza (page 220)	Harley's Potato-Pepper Easy Omelet (page 222)	Herbed Cream Cheese Scramble (page 224)	Red Smoothie (page 186)
Snack 1	C-snack	C-snack	C-snack	C-snack	C-snack
Lunch	Chickpea "Tuna" Salad Sandwich (page 234)	Red Smoothie (page 186)	Smoothie of choice	Quesadilla of choice (page 235)	Chopped Greek Salad (page 260)
Snack 2	C-snack	C-snack	C-snack	C-snack	C-snack
Dinner	Kung Pao-ish Chicken (page 274)	Free meal	10-Minute Stir-Fry (page 276)	Green Soup (page 188)	Free meal

Keep it simple! Last but not least, simplicity is the key to success in dieting, so don't make it harder than it has to be. We have complicated everything in our lives way, way too much. Whenever you haven't succeeded on a diet, I would wager that it's because you overcomplicated it (or, more likely, that the diet itself was overcomplicated to begin with). With the Body Reset Diet, you'll be having a smoothie (or blended soup) a day for the rest of your life—and nothing could be simpler, as you've surely learned by now, than throwing delicious foods into a blender and pressing Start.

Stick to your fitness plan. This is just so, so important, I really can't emphasize it enough. Your fitness plan will be the same as it was during Phase III: as always (do I even need to remind you at this point?), you will keep on walking your 12,000 steps a day, seven days a week. If you're ready to walk even more to expedite the results, then go for it, but do make sure it's a gradual increase. Going too fast is how you get shin splints, plantar fasciitis, and sore knees. It's not so much a problem of repetitive stress injuries as of diminishing returns. In the long run, moderation always wins out.

Don't forget—while physical activity such as walking burns calories, you also have to do regular resistance training to strengthen and tone your body. To that end, you will continue doing Circuit A three days a week and Circuit B two days a week. In general, I'd suggest you make an effort to work out Monday through Friday, but really, any five days will do as long as you're consistent.

As before, you will slowly graduate from the beginner to the intermediate and advanced circuits as your body gets stronger, and once a month you will add an additional circuit to your workout until you reach three circuits. Many of the more advanced exercisers out there who start out doing three circuits will also increase the level of difficulty of the actual exercise. If you start with the more advanced modifications, then keep adding resistance until you feel your body starting to change. My website, www.harleypasternak.com, and my previous books, *The 5-Factor Fitness, The 5-Factor Diet,* and *The 5-Factor World Diet,* are great resources for even more exercises if you feel like you want more variety after several months. Or try my video game, *Harley Pasternak's Hollywood Workout.* Whatever you do, I promise these two simple circuits of four exercises each will transform your body.

The key to all physical activity is being consistent and doing the least you need to do to see the most results. These circuits I've designed are *the* most efficient way of incorporating regular resistance training. I'm not yelling and screaming at you and demanding you do a million completely impossible Olympic feats. I'm asking you to do a tiny series of easy exercises—but do them five days a week, every week, no matter where you are or what else you have going on, so that your body keeps getting better and better.

Keep walking all year round. Not all climates are perfect, and some days walking to work just isn't a feasible option. But you can still get your 12,000 steps in 365 days a year whatever the weather. If it's summer, that might mean getting up early before the heat reaches its peak for your daily stroll. (Or, if you're a night owl, wait till the sun has gone down and get your stroll in later in the evening.) For walks in the middle of the day, bring a bottle of water to keep you cool. In the winter, you're sure to get some good exercise shoveling snow, but that doesn't mean you're off the hook for walking. Stroll up and down the stairs of your office building, or drive to the local mall and power-walk from store to store in between errands. You might have to get a little creative, but I promise it's not that hard to hit 12,000 steps even on the nastiest days of the year!

THE FITNESS BREAKDOWN

Phase I	Phase II	Phase III	The Rest of Your Life
Get an activity tracker. Get a pair of proper-fitting shoes. Walk 10,000 steps/day.	Up your daily step count to 12,000 steps/day. Start a 5-minute resistance circuit (Circuit A), 3 days/week.	Continue to walk 12,000 steps/day. Alternate two resistance circuits (Circuits A and B), 5 days/week.	Continue to walk 12,000 steps/day. Continue alternating Circuits A and B, 5 days/week. Gradually increase to three circuits at every session.

Remember, when it comes to exercise, more is not necessarily better. Think of your body as being like a plant: too little sunlight and it withers up; the same goes for too much sunlight. This exercise regimen is our way of striking the optimal balance between too much and too little resistance training. We want to stimulate our body so that it grows stronger, without overstimulating it so that it gets damaged. Our bodies need time to rest and recover to thrive.

Now . . . pat yourself on the back! As long as you incorporate these lessons into your life, I promise that you will remain successful on the plan, and you will love the dramatic changes in your body. So congratulate yourself on coming this far—and I have all the confidence in the world that you'll continue on this path. Because it works, and when you see how your body changes, you will be inspired to keep going.

Trust me, I know exactly where you're coming from: you want to lose weight ASAP without all the typical roadblocks that have arisen in your years of struggling in vain to lose weight. I heard you loud and clear, and I've designed this plan precisely because I understand how urgent your need is to shed pounds immediately—not next week and not next year, but right away. You came to this book because you've tried everything and nothing has worked for you, whether you're a Hollywood starlet, an executive, or a caregiver. I've seen all the many, many reasons diets don't work, and I've addressed, and offered corrections for every single one of those reasons. I've shown you how to lose weight quickly and easily without sacrificing your health or putting the rest of your life on hold.

This book contains all the answers you need to embrace a healthier—and happier—future, and there's no better moment to start changing your life than right now!

So there you have it: the simplest, safest, and most immediate weight-loss plan ever. And that weight isn't going to come back. I hope this program has taught you how to drop a lot of weight rapidly and—just as important—how to keep it off. You will be amazed at how quickly your body will change, and you definitely won't be the only one who notices!

Appendix A

Glossary of Smoothie Ingredients and Their Benefits

ALMONDS

Expedite weight loss: A 24-week study published in the *International Journal of Obesity* found that low-calorie diets supplemented with almonds, compared to complex carbohydrates, were linked to a 62 percent greater decrease in weight or BMI, a 50 percent greater decrease in waist circumference, and a 56 percent greater decrease in fat mass.[1] Experts believe the heart-healthy monounsaturated fat in almonds helps satisfy the appetite and curb overeating. Researchers at King's College in London found that almonds seem to help stop the absorption of both carbohydrates and the almonds' own fat content into the body, and also that they increased the satisfied feeling of fullness in both men and women.[2]

A 2016 study published in *The Journal of Nutrition* found that eating almonds specifically helped shed belly fat, as well as lower blood pressure.[3]
Improve brainpower: As if almonds need more to recommend them, they also contain phenylalanine, a brain-boosting chemical that aids healthy development of our cognitive functions. A 2017 study published in the *British Journal of Nutrition* found that eating almonds at lunch significantly reduced a post-lunch dip in memory.[4]

APPLES AND PEARS

Expedite weight loss: A Brazilian study found that women who ate three apples or pears per day lost more weight while dieting than women who did not eat fruit while dieting. A 2016 review of several studies found that regular consumption of fruits including apples and pears over a period of four years is associated with a lower body weight; it also found that women randomized to eat apples or pears up to three times a day for 12 weeks lost an average of 2.6 pounds.[5]
Boost the immune system: Red apples contain a powerful antioxidant called quercetin, which can help boost and fortify the immune system, especially when you're stressed out. It's also been shown to be promote resilience in your brain as your age.[6] Quercetin is also found in grapes.
Protect bones: French researchers found that a flavonoid (a type of antioxidant) called phloridzin present only in apples may protect post-menopausal women from osteoporosis and may also increase bone density.[7] Boron, another ingredient in apples, also strengthens bones.

AVOCADOS

Improve the skin: Avocados are Mother Nature's moisturizer. With their healthy fats and phytonutrients, avocados can help prevent wrinkles by keeping the skin moist, soft, and supple.

Boost eye health: Avocados have more of the carotenoid lutein than any other commonly consumed fruit. Lutein protects against macular degeneration and cataracts, two disabling age-related eye diseases.

Improve brain function and memory: Lutein is also protective for the brain. A 2017 study by Tufts University researchers found that when older adults ate one avocado a day for six months, they experienced improved working memory and problem solving skills, as well as increased lutein levels.[8]

Improve satiety: An avocado's fiber and healthy fat content helps you feel fuller, longer. A 2019 study found that when participants ate avocado as part of a meal they felt fuller, even six hours later, than those who hadn't.[9]

Improve nutrient absorption: Avocados contain the antioxidant vitamin E, essential fatty acids, cholesterol-lowering oleic acid, and the heart protectors potassium and folate. But research has also found that, in addition to being filled with nutrients, avocados help us *absorb* nutrients. In one study, when participants ate a salad containing avocados, they absorbed five times the carotenoids (a group of nutrients that includes lycopene and beta-carotene) absorbed by those whose salads didn't include avocados.[10]

BEANS

Keep hunger at bay: Beans are great sources of fiber and protein, both of which are highly satiating. In fact, research has found that beans keep you fuller, longer, even than meat-based protein. Not that I have any problems with animal protein, but it's good to have a variety in your proteins, and beans are no second-best when it comes to keeping you full.

Stabilize blood sugar: Beans are great at keeping your blood sugar levels from spiking. A 2012 study found that Type 2 diabetes patients who added a cup of beans to their daily diet had lower blood sugar and lower blood pressure.[11]

Promote a healthy gut: The fiber in beans feeds the friendly bacteria in your gut, which play a big role in immunity and digestion, helping your whole body function better.

BERRIES

Reduce belly bloat: A University of Michigan Cardiovascular Center study suggests that blueberries may help reduce belly fat and risk factors for cardiovascular disease and metabolic syndrome.[12]

Subtract years: According to a Tufts University study,[13] blueberries are one of nature's most powerful anti-aging supplements. The antioxidant found in blueberries can prevent oxidative damage, a process that damages your cells and ages you.

Improve eyesight: Blueberries' antioxidant properties can prevent or delay age-related eye problems like cataracts and macular degeneration.

BROCCOLI

Protect against cancer: Broccoli, along with other cruciferous vegetables, including cabbage and Brussels sprouts, contains a compound known as indole-3-carbonol, or I3C, that many studies have found to have cancer-fighting abilities—a 2019 study found that I3C works by keeping a tumor-suppressing gene turned on.[14]

Contribute to fat loss: Broccoli is a good source of calcium, and calcium is believed to play a role in the prevention of new fat cells being formed and promoting the breakdown of stored fat.

Builds strong bones: In addition to calcium, broccoli offers a suite of other minerals that work together to create strong bones, including vitamin C, magnesium, and potassium.

CAULIFLOWER

Satisfies a lot of cravings: Cauliflower has become a superstar ingredient because of its versatility—you can roast it and it becomes almost sweet, steam it and mash it with low-fat milk and a little butter and it scratches an itch for mashed potatoes, or eat it raw with hummus when you want something that crunches.

Helps metabolize fat: Cauliflower is a great source of choline, which helps your body do many important things, including process fat. That helps you feel fuller from the fat you eat and less likely to crave more fatty foods.

Protects muscles: Cauliflower is also high in vitamin C (1 cup has 77 percent of the Recommended Daily Allowance), and vitamin C is essential for the formation, maintenance, and repair of muscle tissue. It also boost immunity and helps produce collagen, meaning your stronger all around.

CHIA SEEDS

Expedite weight loss: The essential fatty acids in chia seeds—the survival food of Aztec warriors—help speed up metabolism and promote lean muscle mass. They contain even higher levels of omega-3 fatty acids than salmon and are also high in calcium.

Improve digestion: Chia seeds are also very high in fiber and can add bulk to your diet without adding too many calories. They will help keep food moving through your intestines, which is essential if you want to lose weight.

Help you feel fuller on less food: A 2017 study found that eating at least 7 grams of chia seeds mixed with yogurt lead to consumption of 25 percent fewer calories that day, without feelings of hunger or dips in mood.[15]

CINNAMON

Lowers blood sugar: Studies have shown that the almighty cinnamon can help lower blood sugar in people with diabetes and might also prevent insulin resistance, which leads to diabetes and a host of other health problems, in the rest of the population. Adding cinnamon to a high-carb food might actually lessen the impact of the carbohydrate on your blood sugar levels. It's one of the best metabolism-regulating ingredients there is.

Boosts cognitive function: Cinnamon might help counteract complications associated with traumatic brain injury and stroke that cause restricted blood supply to the brain, according to a study by the U.S. Department of Agriculture.[16] And Alzheimer's disease researchers are currently working to understand the role of cinnamon in alleviating the formation of proteins associated with this ravaging disease of the brain.[17]

GREEK YOGURT, FAT-FREE PLAIN

Expedites weight loss: There's growing evidence that high-calcium diets from dairy sources can aid weight loss. A study published in the *International Journal of Obesity* showed that dieters who ate high-calcium yogurt lost 81 percent more belly fat than dieters on a low-calcium diet. And a University of Tennessee study suggested that dieters who ate three servings of yogurt a day lost 22 percent more weight and 61 percent more body fat than those who simply cut calories and didn't add calcium to their eating plan.

Helps build muscle: A 2019 study found that people who ate nonfat Greek yogurt as part of a 12-week resistance training program gained more strength, bicep muscle thickness, and lean body mass than those who ate a carbohydrate-based placebo.[18]

Improves hair health: Greek yogurt contains a substantial amount of protein, which is important for hair health. If you are vegetarian or just trying to cut back on meat, eating a portion of Greek yogurt may confer the same protein benefits as eating a serving of meat. *U.S. News & World Report* found that 6 ounces of Greek yogurt has about the same amount of protein as 2 to 3 ounces of lean meat, or about 15 to 20 grams. (A comparable serving of regular plain yogurt, the same *U.S. News and World Report* story found, contains only 9 grams of protein, which means you'll be hungrier earlier.)[19]

Provides a great alternative to regular yogurt: Greek yogurt doesn't just beat its conventional counterpart when it comes to protein. It's also lower in lactose and lower in sugar, with a much richer texture and *half* the carbs (5 to 8 grams per serving compared with 13 to 17 grams in regular yogurt)—all for roughly the same calorie count.

LIMES

Fight constipation: The high acid levels in limes, as in all citrus fruits, can have a mild laxative effect and help clean out the bowels. But unlike many citrus fruits, limes are very low in calories—and add tremendous flavor.

Fight disease: Limes are much higher in vitamin C than lemons, which means they have a greater concentration of this essential antioxidant that counteracts free radical damage and protects against a wide range of ailments, from heart disease to cancer.

ORANGES

Protect the immune system: Oranges are rich in vitamin C, a key anti-oxidant that can help protect against immune system deficiencies, cardiovascular disease, prenatal health problems, eye disease, and even skin wrinkling. Vitamin C can even help reverse the free radical damage associated with cancer.

Lower blood pressure: Animal studies have shown that a phytonutrient (or a nutrient found in plants) in oranges, herperidin, can lower both high blood pressure and cholesterol. But this essential ingredient is found only in the peel and white pulp, which means it gets removed during the juicing (but *not* the blending) process.

Promote eye health: A 2018 Australian study followed 2,000 people for 15 years, and found that those who ate at least one serving of oranges every day had more than a 60 percent reduced risk of developing late macular degeneration.[20]

PROTEIN POWDER

Builds healthy muscles and bones: Protein is an essential part of every meal because without it, your body doesn't have the resources to repair itself. Unlike carbohydrates or fats, protein cannot be stored in the body, and it must be frequently consumed. It supplies your body with the essential amino acids it needs to build nails, hair, and muscles.

Helps improve endurance: Whey protein isolate is absorbed quickly into the body and can improve your stamina and endurance during athletic activities, which is one reason professional athletes are such fans of the protein shake. Whey protein also stimulates the release of serotonin, a hormone that promotes feelings of calmness.

Expedites weight loss: The body burns more energy when digesting protein than any other food, and so eating a lot of protein can speed up

Choosing the
Right Protein Powder

Become a label reader when you're shopping for protein powder. Every serving—which should weigh in at 15 to 20 grams—should contain less than 2 grams of fat and 2 grams of sugar. As long as at least 90 percent of the calories come from protein, you're in good shape. But what type of protein powder should you get? The options, I admit, can be dizzying. Here are my favorites, but you can experiment and see which powder works best for you.

- Dairy (whey or casein)
- Egg white (albumin)
- Pea
- Soy (non-GMO)
- Brown rice

your metabolism and help you burn off the pounds. Whey protein can also help slow the absorption rate of glucose into the bloodstream.

SPINACH

Provides great caloric efficiency: Remember when I said that our goal is to make every calorie count? Well, spinach and other leafy green vegetables like kale are among the most calorie-efficient foods you can eat. Spinach contains a wide range of anti-inflammatory and antioxidant agents that can fight everything from osteoporosis to cancer—and all for just 7 calories a cup.

Aids digestion: A single cup of spinach contains nearly 20 percent of the Recommended Dietary Allowance of fiber, meaning it can keep the food moving through your system, fighting constipation and keeping your blood sugar level steady.

Delays aging: Spinach is high in vitamin A, which promotes healthy skin by allowing the epidermis to retain moisture. This in turn can combat psoriasis, acne, wrinkles, and other skin conditions. The high iron and folate content of spinach supports the immune system, enhances vision, slows aging, promotes heart health, and improves blood circulation—all of which can help keep you looking and feeling younger longer.

Strengthens bones: The abundance of vitamin K in spinach helps keep your bones strong, especially as you get older. Vitamin K is also essential for maintaining a healthy nervous system. Basically, if your body needs it done, spinach will do it.

Appendix B

Smoothie Recipes

Basic Recipes

White Smoothie	184
Red Smoothie	186
Green Soup	188

White Smoothies

Apple Pie Smoothie	192
White Peach Ginger Smoothie	193
Tropical Morning Smoothie	194
Pear Spice Smoothie	195
Fall Fruit Frosty	196

Red Smoothies

Ruby Red Frosty	197
Very Berry Smoothie	198
Stonefruit Smoothie	199
PB&J Smoothie	200
Raspberry–Lemon Drop Smoothie	201

Other Smoothies and Soups

Sweet Spinach Smoothie	202
Green Mango Smoothie	203
Kiwi-Strawberry Smoothie	204
Cool Cucumber-Lime Smoothie	205
Caribbean Kale Smoothie	206
Maxwell Mocha Smoothie	207
Piña Colada Smoothie	208
Chocolate Smoothie	209
"Creamy" Cauliflower-Spinach Soup	210
Skinny Mint Pea Soup	211

BASIC RECIPES

White Smoothie

Serves 1

TIPS:
- If your blender isn't powerful enough to grind almonds, you can use chopped almonds or even almond meal instead.
- Be sure to leave the skin on the apple for the fiber boost.
- It's a good idea to buy a couple of extra bananas, peel them, and throw them into the freezer for future smoothies.
- Smoothies blend faster if you add the liquid first. If you like your drinks thinner, feel free to add ice cubes or cold water. This is a great way to increase the volume without adding to your caloric load.

5	raw almonds, whole or chopped
1	red apple, unpeeled, cored and chopped
1	small frozen banana, cut into chunks
¾	cup plain fat-free Greek yogurt
½	cup fat-free milk
½	teaspoon ground cinnamon, or to taste

In a blender or food processer, blend the almonds until finely ground. Add the apple, banana, yogurt, milk, and cinnamon. Blend to desired consistency.

Nutrition Info
Calories: 325
Fat: 4 grams
Carbs: 56 grams
Protein: 19 grams
Fiber: 8 grams

Modified Version (if you weigh more than 175 pounds)

7	raw almonds
1⅓	red apples, unpeeled, cored and chopped
1⅓	small frozen bananas, cut into chunks
1	cup plain fat-free Greek yogurt
¾	cup fat-free milk
¾	teaspoon ground cinnamon, or to taste

Nutrition Info
Calories: 415
Fat: 5 grams
Carbs: 70 grams
Protein: 25 grams
Fiber: 11 grams

SUBSTITUTIONS FOR ALLERGIES & INTOLERANCES

Base Fruit	Accent Flavor
Apple	Cinnamon, to taste
Pear	Ginger, to taste
Peach	Vanilla, to taste

Why These Ingredients?

I devised these recipes with the goal of helping you not only lose weight but also improve your overall health. Every main ingredient has some important health qualities. See Appendix A page 173, for a breakdown of the main ingredients, and an explanation of why they will work wonders on your body.

Red Smoothie

Serves 1

Although nothing beats fresh berries for a snack, frozen fruit is an essential standby for making frosty smoothies year-round. Flash-frozen fruit has the same nutrients as fresh fruit, as long as you choose brands that have no added sugar. (Most don't.) Feel free to mix your berry choices—strawberries and black-berries work just as well. Make sure to use ground flaxseeds rather than whole flaxseeds unless you have a blender that is strong enough to grind the seeds for you.

TIP: You can make this smoothie ahead of time if you prefer. Blend it in the morning, pour the smoothie into a shaker jar, and take it along with you to work. Store in the refrigerator until ready to serve. Add ice as desired and shake well before serving.

- 1   cup frozen raspberries
- ¼   cup frozen blueberries
- ½   orange, peeled and sectioned
- ½   cup cold water, fat-free milk, or nondairy milk
- 1   scoop vanilla protein powder
- 1   tablespoon ground flaxseed

In a blender or food processor, combine the raspberries, blueberries, orange, water, protein powder, and flaxseed. Blend to desired consistency.

Nutrition Info
Calories: 271
Fat: 5 grams
Carbs: 43 grams
Protein: 27 grams
Fiber: 11 grams

Modified Version (if you weigh more than 175 pounds)

1⅓ cups frozen raspberries

½ cup frozen blueberries

½ orange, peeled and sectioned

¾ cup cold water

1⅓ scoops vanilla protein powder

1½ tablespoons ground flaxseed

Nutrition Info
Calories: 325
Fat: 7 grams
Carbs: 55 grams
Protein: 36 grams
Fiber: 14 grams

SUBSTITUTIONS FOR ALLERGIES & INTOLERANCES

BASE FRUIT	FIBER/HEALTHY FAT	PROTEIN
Blueberries/Raspberries	Flaxseeds	Vanilla protein powder
Strawberries	Chia seeds	Other flavor protein powder
Blackberries	Ground walnuts	Fat-free Greek yogurt

Green Soup

It's so easy to eat your vegetables when they've been blended into a tasty soup. You can customize this basic formula by using your favorite vegetable and adding seasonings that will highlight its flavor using the guidelines in the table that follows. I think you'll find that you'll love having this soup even when you're beyond Phase III, or anytime you're feeling like you need an infusion of vegetables—it's easy, warming, and delicious.

TIP: Since you are using only part of the avocado, store the remainder for your next two rounds of green soup. Carve out what you need, then tightly cover the leftover avocado in plastic wrap and refrigerate until you need it again. It will keep for several days in the fridge.

NOTE: This recipe makes two servings—if you're in Phase I, have the first serving at lunch and the second serving for dinner. If you weigh more than 175 pounds, simply increase your portion of protein—it should weigh about as much as the mass of your hand.

2	cups water
1½	cups prepared vegetables (see chart at right)
1	bouillon cube
¼	ripe avocado
	Seasoning (see chart or simply use salt and pepper to taste)
2	(3- to 4-ounce) pieces prepared protein of choice (grilled chicken, steamed shrimp, salmon, or tofu; see page 190)

In a medium pot, bring the water to a boil. Add the veggies and cook according to the time given in the chart, until the color is vibrant and the vegetables are just tender. Transfer the veggies and cooking water (it contains vitamins that leached from the veggies during cooking) to a blender along with bouillon cube, avocado, and seasoning and blend until smooth and creamy. Transfer to bowls and top with the protein of choice or serve the protein on the side.

Modified Version (if you weigh more than 175 pounds)

2⅓ cups water

2   cups prepared vegetables

1   bouillon cube

½   ripe avocado

      Seasoning

2   (4- to 6-ounce) pieces prepared protein of choice

Vegetable	Preparation	Cook time	Seasoning Suggestions
Asparagus	Tough ends removed, cut into bite-sized pieces	2–3 minutes	¼ cup fresh parsley, zest of 1 lemon, ½ tsp. black pepper
Broccoli	Cut into florets	4–5 minutes	½ tsp. garlic powder, ¼ tsp. dried oregano, drizzle with balsamic vinegar before serving
Spinach (or other leafy green)	Increase amount by 1 cup; tear into bite-sized pieces, remove any tough stems	2–3 minutes	¼ tsp. each garlic powder and onion powder, zest of 1 lemon
Zucchini	Cut into bite-sized pieces	6–7 minutes	1 tsp. dried basil, ½ tsp. each garlic powder and onion powder

For 175 lbs and less	For 175 lbs and over
Calories: 230	Calories: 361
Fat: 8 grams	Fat: 14 grams
Carbs: 12 grams	Carbs: 167 grams
Protein: 27 grams	Protein: 40 grams
Fiber: 5 grams	Fiber: 7 grams

For the protein (per serving):

Chicken: Lightly salt a 3- to 4-ounce piece of boneless, skinless chicken breast. Set on a plate while bringing a skillet or grill pan to medium-high heat. Lightly brush (or spray) the pan with oil and pat chicken dry. Sear chicken 3 to 4 minutes per side, until golden brown. Then, pour ¼ cup water into the pan, turn the heat to medium low, and simmer 6 to 9 minutes, until a thermometer inserted into the thickest part of the meat reads 165°F. Another great option is to use 3 to 4 ounces of sliced grocery-store rotisserie chicken. I like to portion out the meat when I bring these rotisserie chickens home so I always have just the right amount.

Shrimp: In a skillet, heat ½ cup water, a pinch of salt, and (if you have it) a sliced lemon. Add 3 to 4 ounces of frozen peeled shrimp, and cook over medium heat until the shrimp are pink, firm, and cooked through, 7 to 8 minutes. You can also use frozen cooked shrimp. Just thaw completely to enjoy cold or cook until just warmed through, 3 minutes.

Salmon: Lightly salt the flesh side of a 3- to 4-ounce piece of skin-on salmon fillet. Bring a skillet to medium-high heat. Lightly brush (or spray) the pan with oil and pat salmon dry. Sear skin side down for 7 to 8 minutes, until skin easily releases from pan (if it's not letting go, it's not ready). Flip, and cook an additional 2 to 3 minutes, skin side up, until a thermometer inserted into the thickest part of the salmon reads 130°F or until the fish flakes easily with a fork. For an even simpler option, use flaked smoked salmon instead.

Tofu: Chop 3 to 4 ounces of extra-firm tofu into bite-sized pieces, then lay on a paper towel–lined plate. Put another paper towel on top, then a plate. Press down to extract moisture from the tofu. Bring a skillet to medium-high heat. Warm a teaspoon of oil, then add the tofu carefully (it might spatter). Cook, stirring frequently, until tofu is golden brown on all sides, about 5 minutes. Season with salt and pepper before serving.

Congratulations! You've just completed your first day of Phase I—and you've learned how to make simple, nutritious meals for the rest of your life. You'll find plenty of alternative smoothie and blended soup recipes starting on the next page.

"As a working mom of four kids (two of them with special needs), I would LOVE to tell other busy women that weight loss and health are just around the corner for them if they want them badly enough. They just need to take it one day at a time and realize that taking care of themselves is NOT selfish. On the contrary, it's the most loving gift they can give to their loved ones. If I can do it with all my time constraints (and my own physical limitations), then anyone can!"

—MERCEDES J., LOST 13 POUNDS IN 15 DAYS

WHITE SMOOTHIES

NOTE: If you weigh more than 175 pounds, modify these recipes by using one-third more of each ingredient.

Apple Pie Smoothie   Serves 1

Be sure to leave the skin on the apple for the added fiber. It's a good idea to buy a couple of extra bananas and throw them in the freezer for future smoothies.

TIP: If you like your drinks thinner, feel free to add ice cubes or cold water.

5	raw almonds
1	red apple, unpeeled, cored and chopped
1	small frozen banana, chopped
6	ounces plain fat-free Greek yogurt
½	cup fat-free or nondairy milk
½	teaspoon ground cinnamon, or to taste

In a blender or food processer, blend the almonds until finely ground. Add the apple, banana, yogurt, milk, and cinnamon. Blend to desired consistency.

Nutrition Info
Calories: 325
Fat: 4 grams
Carbs: 56 grams
Protein: 19 grams
Fiber: 8 grams

White Peach Ginger Smoothie

Serves 1

Remember, the riper the fruit, the sweeter the smoothie. If peaches are in season, select the ripest you can find at the market. If not, use frozen peaches.

TIP: Just for fun, the raspberries aren't blended in this drink. Instead, they are dropped into the glass; serve this drink with a spoon for scooping up the berries.

- 2   peaches, pitted and chopped
- 6   ounces plain fat-free Greek yogurt
- 2   tablespoons fresh lime juice
- ½   teaspoon finely chopped peeled fresh ginger, or pinch of ground ginger
- ½ to ¾ cup water, or ½ cup fat-free or nondairy milk
- ½   cup fresh raspberries
- 10 pistachios (unsalted), shelled, crushed or coarsely chopped

In a blender or food processor, combine the peaches, yogurt, lime juice, and ginger. Add the water and blend to desired consistency. Pour into a tall serving glass. Gently stir in the raspberries and garnish with the pistachios.

Nutrition Info
Calories: 300
Fat: 2 grams
Carbs: 41 grams
Protein: 27 grams
Fiber: 9 grams

Tropical Morning Smoothie

Serves 1

Greek yogurt provides almost double the protein of regular yogurt. That and its super-creamy texture make it an ideal addition to a healthy smoothie. However, if you can't find it, feel free to substitute regular plain yogurt—if you want to make it have a similar, thicker texture like Greek yogurt, you can strain it either in a fine mesh strainer or in a colander that's been lined with cheesecloth for 30 minutes or so, but it's not necessary. (Avoid vanilla yogurt, as it's loaded with added sugar.)

TIP: Opt for fresh pineapple over canned for this recipe.

- ½ cup fresh or frozen mango chunks
- ½ cup fresh pineapple chunks
- 1 frozen banana, chopped
- 6 ounces plain fat-free Greek yogurt
- 2 tablespoons ground flaxseed
- ½ to ¾ cup water, or ½ cup fat-free or nondairy milk

In a blender or food processor, combine the mango, pineapple, banana, yogurt, and flaxseed. Add the water and blend to desired consistency.

Nutrition Info
Calories: 300
Fat: 6 grams
Carbs: 38 grams
Protein: 22 grams
Fiber: 8 grams

Pear Spice Smoothie Serves 1

This drink is especially good in the fall, when pears are seasonal.

TIP: Experiment with the different types of protein powders. Once you've found one you like, you can save money by purchasing it in bulk.

- 1   pear, unpeeled, cored and chopped
- 1   frozen banana, chopped
- 1   teaspoon finely chopped peeled fresh ginger, or pinch of ground ginger
-     Pinch of ground cinnamon
-     Pinch of grated nutmeg
- 2   tablespoons unflavored protein powder or vanilla extract
- ½   cup ice cubes or crushed ice
- ½   to ¾ cup water, or ½ cup fat-free or nondairy milk

In a blender or food processor, combine the pear, banana, ginger, cinnamon, nutmeg, protein powder, and ice. Add the water and blend to desired consistency.

Nutrition Info
Calories: 300
Fat: 2 grams
Carbs: 55 grams
Protein: 25 grams
Fiber: 10 grams

Fall Fruit Frosty

Serves 1

The familiar flavors of this mild smoothie will please the whole family.

TIP: Yogurt is often sold in 6-ounce containers, which is why that size is specified in these smoothie recipes. If you make a lot of smoothies, you can certainly buy a bigger container and use ¾ cup measure for the 6 ounces.

1   green apple, unpeeled, cored and chopped

1   ripe green pear (such as green Anjou or Bartlett pears), unpeeled, cored and chopped

6   ounces plain fat-free Greek yogurt

2   teaspoons creamy-style peanut butter

1   cup small ice cubes or crushed ice

½ to ¾ cup water, or ½ cup fat-free or nondairy milk

In a blender or food processor, combine the apple, pear, yogurt, peanut butter, and ice. Add the water and blend to desired consistency.

Nutrition Info
Calories: 300
Fat: 4 grams
Carbs: 52 grams
Protein: 18 grams
Fiber: 10 grams

RED SMOOTHIES

NOTE: If you weigh more than 175 pounds, modify these recipes by using one-third more of each ingredient.

Ruby Red Frosty

Serves 1

Although nothing beats fresh berries for a snack, reach for frozen fruit to make frosty smoothies year-round. Feel free to mix your berry choices—strawberries and blackberries work just as well. Make sure to use ground flaxseed rather than whole flaxseeds.

TIP: Make the smoothie ahead of time. Pour it into a shaker jar and store it in the refrigerator until you're ready to enjoy it. Add ice as desired and shake well before serving.

- 1 cup frozen raspberries
- ¼ cup frozen blueberries
- ½ orange, peeled and sectioned
- 2 tablespoons unflavored protein powder or vanilla extract
- 1 tablespoon ground flaxseed
- ½ to ¾ cup water, or ½ cup fat-free or nondairy milk

In a blender or food processor, combine the raspberries, blueberries, orange, protein powder, and flaxseed. Add the water and blend to desired consistency.

Nutrition Info
Calories: 270
Fat: 5 grams
Carbs: 34 grams
Protein: 27 grams
Fiber: 11 grams

Very Berry Smoothie

Serves 1

Feel free to vary the berry with the season for this sweet treat. Nothing in season? Frozen berries work perfectly!

TIP: Blending a whole orange rather than using just the juice means you'll get all the fiber and vitamins from the orange, with none of the fillers or sugar that juices sometimes contain.

- ¾ cup fresh or frozen raspberries
- ¾ cup fresh or frozen pitted cherries
- ½ to ¾ cup fat-free or nondairy milk
- 1 orange, peeled and sectioned
- 2 tablespoons unflavored protein powder or vanilla extract

In a blender or food processor, combine the raspberries, cherries, milk, orange, and protein powder. Blend to desired consistency.

Nutrition Info
Calories: 275
Fat: 5 grams
Carbs: 42 grams
Protein: 21 grams
Fiber: 10 grams

Stonefruit Smoothie Serves 1

In most instances, we prefer fresh fruit to frozen. For smoothies, however, frozen fruit adds a refreshing icy texture to the drink.

TIP: If the peaches at your market are mealy, reach for frozen instead. No apricots? Throw in an extra half a peach.

- 2 ripe peaches, pitted and chopped
- 1 ripe apricot, pitted and chopped
- 1 cup fresh or frozen strawberries
- 6 ounces plain fat-free Greek yogurt
- 2 tablespoons ground flaxseed
- 1 cup small ice cubes or crushed ice
- ½ to ¾ cup water, or ½ cup fat-free milk or nondairy milk

In a blender or food processor, combine the peaches, apricot, strawberries, yogurt, flaxseed, and ice. Add the water and blend to desired consistency.

Nutrition Info
Calories: 310
Total Fat: 7 grams
Carbs: 46 grams
Protein: 20 grams
Fiber: 11 grams

PB&J Smoothie

Serves 1

Your favorite sandwich flavors can be transformed into a satisfying midday drink.

TIP: Got overripe berries or fruits? Don't throw them out; instead, freeze them for smoothies. Prep and chop the fruit so it's ready to use later; you can just throw it all into the same bag.

2   cups chopped fresh or frozen strawberries

1   frozen banana, chopped

2   teaspoons creamy peanut butter

4   ounces plain fat-free Greek yogurt, or ½ cup fat-free milk

½   cup ice cubes or crushed ice

In a blender or food processor, combine the strawberries, banana, peanut butter, yogurt, and ice. Blend to desired consistency.

Nutrition Info
Calories: 310
Fat: 7 grams
Carbs: 47 grams
Protein: 17 grams
Fiber: 9 grams

Raspberry–Lemon Drop Smoothie

Serves 1

Just for fun, garnish your glass with a twist of lemon peel.

TIP: Too busy to juice the lemons? Look for pure lemon juice in the refrigerator section of your supermarket.

1   cup frozen raspberries

12 raw cashews

3   tablespoons fresh lemon juice

6   ounces plain fat-free Greek yogurt

¾ cup ice cubes or crushed ice

½ teaspoon grated lemon peel (optional)

½ to ¾ cup water, or ½ cup fat-free or nondairy milk

In a blender or food processor, combine the raspberries, cashews, lemon juice, yogurt, ice, and lemon peel, if using. Add the water and blend to desired consistency.

Nutrition Info
Calories: 274
Fat: 9 grams
Carbs: 31 grams
Protein: 21 grams
Fiber: 10 grams

OTHER SMOOTHIES AND SOUPS

NOTE: If you weigh more than 175 pounds, modify these recipes by using one-third more of each ingredient.

Sweet Spinach Smoothie

Serves 1

A spinach smoothie is a great way to add leafy greens to your diet. Here, spinach is paired with sweet grapes and pears, creamy yogurt, avocado, and a splash of lime juice.

TIP: Since you are using only part of the avocado, carve out what's needed here, then tightly cover the remaining avocado with plastic wrap and refrigerate until you need it again.

- 2 cups (packed) fresh spinach leaves
- 1 ripe pear, peeled, cored, and chopped
- 15 green or red grapes
- 6 ounces plain fat-free Greek yogurt
- 2 tablespoons chopped avocado
- 1 to 2 tablespoons fresh lime juice
- ½ to ¾ cup water, or ½ cup fat-free or nondairy milk

In a blender or food processor, combine the spinach, pear, grapes, yogurt, avocado, and lime juice to taste. Add the water and blend to desired consistency.

Nutrition Info
Calories: 315
Fat: 7 grams
Carbs: 43 grams
Protein: 25 grams
Fiber: 9 grams

Green Mango Smoothie

Serves 1

Although we feature chard in this drink, you can always substitute spinach, kale, or any other dark leafy green.

TIP: Remember to trim the chard before adding it to the blender. The thick woody stems are too tough to include in the smoothie.

1½ cups chopped fresh chard

1   cup fresh or frozen mango chunks

½   cup fresh or frozen blueberries

2   tablespoons unflavored protein powder

½   cup ice cubes or crushed ice

½   to ¾ cup water, or ½ cup fat-free or nondairy milk

In a blender or food processor, combine the chard, mango, blueberries, protein powder, and ice. Add the water and blend to desired consistency.

Nutrition Info
Calories: 320
Fat: 2 grams
Carbs: 64 grams
Protein: 20 grams
Fiber: 9 grams

Kiwi-Strawberry Smoothie

Serves 1

Baby arugula adds a peppery bite to this refreshing drink. These delicate, tiny leaves are a super-flexible ingredient; they're delicious eaten fresh in salads, cooked as a side dish, or swirled into a smoothie.

TIP: In general, it's good to include the skins of fruits like apples, peaches, and pears in your smoothies to up the fiber content. For this smoothie, though, you need to peel the kiwi fruit; that skin is too tough.

2   cups baby arugula

2   kiwifruits, peeled and chopped

5   fresh or frozen strawberries, chopped

1   frozen banana, chopped

2   tablespoons protein powder

½ to ¾ cup water, or ½ cup fat-free or nondairy milk

In a blender or food processor, combine the arugula, kiwifruits, strawberries, banana, and protein powder. Add the water and blend to desired consistency.

Nutrition Info
Calories: 300
Fat: 3 grams
Carbs: 54 grams
Protein: 21 grams
Fiber: 9 grams

Cool Cucumber-Lime Smoothie

Serves 1

1   small cucumber, peeled

1   tablespoon fresh lime juice

10 frozen green grapes

6   ounces plain fat-free Greek yogurt

½   cup ice cubes or crushed ice

½ to ¾ cup water, or ½ cup fat-free or nondairy milk

Fresh mint leaf, for garnish (optional)

In a blender or food processor, combine the cucumber, lime juice, grapes, yogurt, and ice. Add the water and blend to desired consistency. Garnish with the mint leaf, if desired.

Nutrition Info
Calories: 320
Fat: 1 gram
Carbs: 63 grams
Protein: 22 grams
Fiber: 6 grams

Caribbean Kale Smoothie

Serves 1

Coconut extract adds a taste of the tropics to this satisfying drink.

TIP: For greater ease in blending, use crushed ice.

- 1   cup chopped fresh kale leaves
- 1   small frozen banana, chopped
- 1   cup frozen mango chunks
- 2   tablespoons unflavored protein powder
- ½   teaspoon coconut extract
- 1   cup ice cubes or crushed ice
- ½ to ¾ cup water, or ½ cup fat-free or nondairy milk

In a blender or food processor, combine the kale, banana, mango, protein powder, coconut extract, and ice. Add the water and blend to desired consistency.

Nutrition Info
Calories: 310
Fat: 2 grams
Carbs: 56 grams
Protein: 26 grams
Fiber: 9 grams

Maxwell Mocha Smoothie

Serves 1

As refreshing as a frappuccino, without the mountains of added sugar.

TIP: For greater ease in blending, use crushed ice.

- 2 tablespoons chocolate whey powder
- 2 teaspoons chia seed powder
- 1 cup almond milk
- 2 to 4 tablespoons espresso, cooled
- 1 tablespoon stevia
- 1 cup ice cubes or crushed ice

In a blender or food processor, combine the whey powder, chia seed powder, almond milk, espresso, stevia and ice. Blend to desired consistency.

Piña Colada Smoothie

There's no reason why eating healthy can't feel festive! Transport yourself to a beachside resort with these tropical tastes.

TIP: Use fresh pineapple for this, not canned.

- 1   medium orange, peeled and sectioned
- ⅓   cup coconut milk
- 2   tablespoons whey protein powder
- 1   frozen banana, chopped
- 1   cup fresh pineapple chunks

In a blender or food processor, combine the orange, coconut milk, protein powder, banana, and pineapple. Blend to desired consistency. Paper umbrella optional.

Chocolate Smoothie

Serves 1

This chocolaty drink is a great, healthy way to satisfy a sweet tooth.

TIP: Stevia comes as either a powder or a liquid. Since it's a lot sweeter than sugar (without any impact on your blood sugar!), add it a little at a time until you find the right level for your taste. A little goes a long way.

- 1   frozen banana, chopped
- 2   tablespoons unsweetened cocoa powder
- 2   tablespoons whey protein powder
- 1   cup almond milk
- ½   teaspoon stevia or other sweetener
- 5   whole almonds

In a blender or food processor, combine the banana, cocoa powder, protein powder, almond milk, stevia, and almonds. Blend to desired consistency.

Nutrition Info
Calories: 284
Fat: 7 grams
Carbs: 38 grams
Protein: 27 grams
Fiber: 7 grams

"Creamy" Cauliflower-Spinach Soup

Serves 2

Blending the cauliflower gives it a creamy consistency; spinach keeps this soup green.

TIP: You can store the leftovers in a bowl, covered in plastic wrap, in the fridge. When you're ready to serve, simply give it a stir and warm it in the microwave.

- 2 cups water
- ¾ cup cauliflower florets
- 2 cups baby spinach leaves
- 1 bouillon cube
- ½ ripe avocado
- ½ teaspoon each ground turmeric, ground cumin, and paprika
- 2 (3- to 4-ounce) prepared servings protein of choice (grilled chicken, steamed shrimp, salmon, or tofu; see page 190)

Place the water in a medium pot and bring to a boil. Add the cauliflower and cook 4 to 5 minutes, until just tender. Add the spinach and cook 1 to 2 minutes, until wilted. Transfer the vegetables and cooking water to a blender. Add the bouillon cube, avocado, and seasonings, and blend until smooth and creamy. Pour into serving bowls and top with the protein choice or serve the protein on the side.

Nutrition Info
Calories: 300
Fat: 14 grams
Carbs: 9 grams
Protein: 36 grams
Fiber: 5 grams

Skinny Mint Pea Soup

Serves 2

I always have a bag of green peas in the freezer—this soup is refreshing any time of year.

TIP: Mint is super easy to grow; get a small pot to put on your windowsill or grow it in a planter outside—just don't put it in your garden, as mint will spread and crowd out your other plants.

- 2   cups water
- 1½ cups frozen peas
- 1   bouillon cube
- ½   ripe avocado
- 3   to 4 fresh mint leaves
- ¼   teaspoon garlic powder
- ¼   teaspoon onion powder
- 2   (3- to 4-ounce) prepared servings protein of choice (grilled chicken, steamed shrimp, salmon, or tofu; see page 190)

Place the water in a medium pot and bring to a boil. Add the peas and cook 2 to 3 minutes, until just tender. Transfer the peas and water to a blender. Add the bouillon cube, avocado, and seasonings and blend until smooth and creamy.

Pour into serving bowls and top with the protein or serve the protein on the side.

Nutrition Info
Calories: 376
Fat: 14 grams
Carbs: 23 grams
Protein: 41 grams
Fiber: 10 grams

Appendix C

C-Snack Guidelines

Remember, these snacks should be crunchy and contain a protein. They should all be about 150 calories and have at least 5 grams of fiber, 5 grams of protein, and less than 10 grams of sugar. You can feel free to mix and match, but here are some ideas for both complete snacks and satisfying combos.

Complete Snacks

Air-popped popcorn
Soy nuts (roasted soybeans)
Freeze-dried peas
Crunchsters (made from sprouted mung beans)

Combo Snacks

1½ bags Cruncha Ma-Me
—135 calories, 12 grams protein, 5 grams fiber

⅔ cup fresh raspberries + 8 ounces fat-free Greek yogurt
—170 calories, 23 grams protein, 6 grams fiber

4 Finn Crisp crackers + 2 slices Kraft fat-free cheese
—170 calories, 18 grams protein, 5 grams fiber

½ cup fat-free cottage cheese + ½ cup Fiber One cereal + ¼ cup
   fresh blueberries
—160 calories, 15 grams protein, 15 grams fiber

⅓ cup fat-free Greek yogurt + ⅓ tablespoon natural peanut butter +
   1 Gala apple
—160 calories, 10 grams protein, 6 grams fiber

3 slices turkey breast + 3 Ryvita crackers + 1 teaspoon mustard
—153 calories, 14 grams protein, 5 grams fiber

1 large Bosc pear + 1 low-fat cheese stick
—170 calories, 9 grams protein, 4 grams fiber

¾ cup cooked edamame
—143 calories, 13 grams protein, 6 grams fiber

3 ounces lean roast beef + 1½ red bell peppers
—155 calories, 19 grams protein, 5 grams fiber

1 tall Starbucks latte with fat-free milk + 1 apple
—154 calories, <1 gram protein, 2.4 grams fiber

5 celery ribs + 1 tablespoon natural peanut butter
—155 calories, 7 grams protein, 6 grams fiber

2 whole-grain Ryvita crackers + 3 tablespoons hummus
—140 calories, 5 grams protein, 6 grams fiber

1 apple + 3 turkey slices
—155 calories, 11 grams protein, 5 grams fiber

1 pear + 2 ounces sliced lean roast beef
—165 calories, 14 grams protein, 5 grams fiber

1 cucumber + 3 ounces smoked salmon + 1 ripe tomato
—165 calories, 19 grams protein, 4 grams fiber

3 Finn Crisp crackers + 1 tablespoon almond butter
—155 calories, 5 grams protein, 5 grams fiber

2 slices Kraft fat-free cheese + 3 Kavli Golden Rye crispbreads
—140 calories, 11 grams protein, 6 grams fiber

2 triangles Laughing Cow Light cheese + 5 Grissol multi-grain
    melba toast crackers
—170 calories, 7 grams protein, 5 grams fiber

Appendix D

S-Meal Recipes

Scrambles 218

Sandwiches 233

Soups 246

Salads 258

Stir-Fries 272

SCRAMBLES

If you like, you can substitute a whole egg for one of the egg whites after the first 15 days. Just remember that doing so will add more fat and calories to the meal.

Onion, Turkey Sausage, and Spinach Frittata

Serves 6

Cook this once and you'll have plenty of leftovers to get you through a busy week. It's good served cold or rewarmed.

- 2 tablespoons olive oil
- 1 large yellow onion, thinly sliced
- 3 links fresh Italian-flavored turkey sausage, sliced
- 1 (6-ounce) bag baby spinach
  Salt and black pepper
- 3 large eggs
- 1⅓ cups liquid egg whites
- ⅔ cup fat-free or low-fat milk

1. Preheat the oven to 325ºF.
2. In a large oven-safe skillet (such as cast iron), heat the olive oil over medium heat. Add the onion and sauté 2 to 3 minutes, until onion begins to be translucent. Add the sausage, and sauté 3 to 5 more minutes, until onion is tender and the sausage is cooked through.
3. Add the spinach and a small pinch of salt and cook for 3 minutes, stirring frequently, until the spinach is wilted and any liquid that has been released is evaporated. Remove the skillet from the heat and let cool.
4. Whisk together the eggs, egg whites, milk, and salt and pepper until blended and frothy. Pour the egg mixture over the spinach mixture, and transfer the skillet to the oven.
5. Bake for 25 to 35 minutes, until the eggs are just set and are pulling away from the sides of the pan. Slice and serve.

Nutrition Info
Calories: 158
Fat: 10 grams
Carbs: 5 grams
Protein: 12 grams
Fiber: 1 gram

Italian Flag Breakfast Pizza

Serves 1

For the fluffiest scramble, give the egg whites a good strong whisk before adding them to the pan.

TIP: It's okay to pile the spinach high—it will wilt.

	Nonstick cooking spray
3	egg whites, or 6 tablespoons liquid egg substitute
	Salt and black pepper
3	cherry tomatoes, cut into halves
1	whole wheat pita bread
1	cup baby spinach
1	ounce part-skim mozzarella cheese, shredded

1. Preheat the broiler. Line a baking pan with foil. Place the pan under the broiler to warm it. Coat a small nonstick skillet with cooking spray and place it over medium-high heat.

2. In a small bowl, whisk together the egg whites, salt, and pepper. Pour into the skillet and cook for 30 seconds, stirring constantly. Remove from the heat and stir in the tomatoes.

3. Remove the baking pan from the oven. Place the pita on the baking pan and top with the spinach, then add the egg mixture and the cheese. Season to taste with additional salt and pepper.

4. Broil for 2 minutes, or until the eggs are set and the pita is golden.

Nutrition Info
Calories: 320
Fat: 7 grams
Carbs: 37 grams
Protein: 26 grams
Fiber: 7 grams

Harley's Potato-Pepper Easy Omelet

Serves 1

Omelets the easy way! Use a rubber spatula to push and form the omelet in the pan as it cooks—no tricky folding required.

TIP: Leave the skin on the potato for added flavor. Just be sure to use a boiling (waxy) potato, not a baking potato.

	Nonstick cooking spray
1	waxy potato, such as Yukon Gold, halved and thinly sliced
½	red bell pepper, thinly sliced
½	small onion, thinly sliced
	Salt and black pepper
5	egg whites, or 10 tablespoons liquid egg substitute
1	tablespoon shredded Cheddar cheese
1	slice double-fiber whole wheat bread

1. Coat a small nonstick skillet with cooking spray and place it over medium heat. Add the potato, bell pepper, and onion and season with the salt and pepper. Cook for 8 to 10 minutes, stirring frequently, until the vegetables soften and are lightly browned.

2. Pour the egg whites into the skillet, gently coating the vegetable mixture with them. Using a spatula, press down on the omelet to flatten it as it cooks. Cook for 1 minute, or until just set. Use the spatula to fold the omelet in half and push it to one-half of the pan, forming a half-moon shape. Sprinkle the top with the cheese. Cover the skillet for 30 seconds to melt the cheese.

3. Toast the bread.

4. Slide the omelet onto a serving plate. Season to taste with additional salt and pepper. Serve the omelet with the toast.

Nutrition Info
Calories: 355
Fat: 5 grams
Carbs: 57 grams
Protein: 29 grams
Fiber: 12 grams

Herbed Cream Cheese Scramble

Serves 1

This creamy scramble cooks in seconds, making it a perfect workday morning meal.

TIP: Smoked salmon has such an intense flavor that you need only a small amount!

1	ounce reduced-fat cream cheese, at room temperature
1	tablespoon chopped fresh dill
1	tablespoon chopped fresh chives
	Salt
	Nonstick cooking spray
4	egg whites, or ½ cup liquid egg substitute
	Black pepper
2	slices double-fiber whole wheat bread
2	ounces smoked salmon, julienned

1. In a small bowl, mash the cream cheese, dill, and chives until blended and smooth. Stir in a pinch of salt.
2. Coat a small skillet with cooking spray and place over medium heat.
3. In a small bowl, whisk the egg whites, additional salt, and some pepper. Cook the egg mixture, stirring frequently, for 2 to 3 minutes, until almost set.
4. Toast the bread.
5. Remove the scrambled eggs from the heat. Fold in the reserved cream cheese mixture and the salmon. Serve with the toast.

Nutrition Info
Calories: 300
Fat: 9 grams
Carbs: 32 grams
Protein: 33 grams
Fiber: 14 grams

Sweet Potato Hash with Chives

Serves 1

Hearty, healthy, homey—a perfect winter weather breakfast.

TIP: For quick cooking, it's important to cut the potato and bell pepper into small cubes.

1   sweet potato, peeled and finely chopped
    Nonstick cooking spray
1   small onion, chopped
1   red bell pepper, cored, seeded, and finely chopped
    Salt and black pepper
4   egg whites, or ½ cup liquid egg substitute
½   teaspoon ground paprika
    Fresh chives, for garnish

1. In a shallow microwave-safe bowl, place the sweet potatoes and just enough water to cover. Cover the bowl and microwave on high power for 4 minutes, or until the sweet potatoes are tender. Drain.

2. Coat a large nonstick skillet with cooking spray and place it over medium heat. Add the onion, bell pepper, and the sweet potatoes. Season with the salt and pepper and cook for 5 minutes, stirring frequently, until tender. Increase the heat to medium high and cook for 5 more minutes, until crisp. Scrape the hash onto a serving plate and cover it to keep it warm.

3. In a small bowl, whisk the egg whites. Add the beaten egg whites to the hot skillet and reduce the heat to medium. Quickly scramble the eggs for 2 to 3 minutes, to desired doneness.

4. Spoon the eggs atop the hash. Season to taste with additional salt and pepper and the paprika. Garnish with the chives.

Nutrition Info
Calories: 340
Fat: 3 grams
Carbs: 60 grams
Protein: 23 grams
Fiber: 12 grams

Harley's Hearty Egg Muffin

Serves 1

A fast-food dish takes on a healthier profile by using whole wheat muffins and egg whites and adding savory mushrooms.

TIP: Fresh thyme is a nice addition to the mushrooms, but if you don't have any, the dish is still delicious without it.

	Nonstick cooking spray
2	tablespoons chopped shallot or onion
5	white button mushrooms, sliced
	Salt and black pepper
	Minced fresh thyme
4	egg whites, or ½ cup liquid egg substitute
1	whole wheat English muffin
2	tablespoons shredded Cheddar cheese

1. Coat a small nonstick skillet with cooking spray and place it over medium–low heat. Add the shallot and mushrooms and cook for 4 minutes, stirring frequently, until the mushrooms give off their juices and are softened. Season to taste with the salt, pepper, and thyme. Scrape the mixture into a bowl.

2. Coat the same skillet with additional cooking spray and place it over medium heat. In a bowl, whisk the egg whites, then add to the skillet. Scramble the egg whites for 2 to 3 minutes, until they are set.

3. Toast the English muffin.

4. On a serving plate, top each muffin half with half the eggs and half the mushroom mixture. Sprinkle with the cheese and cover briefly with foil to melt the cheese, then serve.

Nutrition Info
Calories: 290
Fat: 7 grams
Carbs: 35 grams
Protein: 28 grams
Fiber: 7 grams

Breakfast Burritos I Serves 2

*Burritos are my favorite "on the go" breakfast. They are very
filling and easy to make.*

Nonstick cooking spray

5 white button mushrooms, sliced

2 egg whites, or ¼ cup liquid egg substitute

1 teaspoon onion powder

2 teaspoons taco seasoning mix

Salt and cracked black peppercorns

1 cup fat-free ricotta

2 whole-grain or whole wheat tortillas

2 cups diced ripe tomatoes

2 cups spinach leaves

1. Coat a medium nonstick skillet with cooking spray and place it over
   medium heat. Add the mushrooms and cook for 2 minutes, until they turn
   golden. Add the egg whites, onion powder, taco seasoning mix, and salt
   and pepper to taste. Stir in the ricotta and cook for 1 minute, stirring
   frequently, until the eggs are fully cooked. Keep warm.
2. Microwave each tortilla on high for 20 seconds, then place it on a cutting
   board. Place some of the scrambled eggs, the tomatoes, and spinach on
   each tortilla. Roll tightly into a burrito shape. Slice each burrito in half
   and serve.

Nutrition Info
Calories: 374
Fat: 4 grams
Carbs: 56 grams
Protein: 34 grams
Fiber: 11 grams

Breakfast Burritos II Serves 2

Living in L.A., I've learned to love Mexican food. This is my
healthy spin on an egg burrito.

> Nonstick cooking spray
>
> 16 egg whites, or 2 cups liquid egg substitute
>
> Salt and black pepper
>
> 2 large whole-grain or whole wheat tortillas
>
> 1¼ cups refried beans, warmed
>
> ¼ cup shredded fat-free Cheddar cheese
>
> 2 cups mild or spicy salsa

1. Coat a medium nonstick skillet with cooking spray and place it over medium heat. Pour in the egg whites and salt and pepper and cook, stirring frequently, for 1½ minutes, until the eggs are cooked through. Keep warm.
2. Microwave the tortillas on high power for 15 seconds. Spread the refried beans on the tortillas and spoon the scrambled eggs over them. Sprinkle the cheese on top and roll the tortillas tightly into a burrito shape.
3. Cut each burrito in half. Spoon the salsa over the burritos or serve on the side.

Nutrition Info
Calories: 465
Fat: 3 grams
Carbs: 62 grams
Protein: 46 grams
Fiber: 15 grams

Sweet Potato Home Fries and Eggs

Serves 2

Like your typical diner breakfast—only healthier!

TIP: If fat-free Cheddar cheese is difficult to find, replace it with shredded part-skim mozzarella.

1¼ pounds sweet potatoes (about 2 medium)

Nonstick cooking spray

½ cup finely chopped Spanish onion

2 bell peppers, cored, seeded, and finely chopped

1 teaspoon ground paprika

1½ teaspoons garlic powder

1 teaspoon red pepper flakes

8 egg whites, or 1 cup liquid egg substitute

1 cup shredded fat-free Cheddar cheese (4 ounces)

Salt and cracked black peppercorns

1. Microwave the sweet potatoes on high power for 3 minutes. Let cool somewhat, then peel and finely chop.

2. Coat a large nonstick pan with cooking spray and place it over medium heat. Add the onion and cook for 1 minute, stirring frequently, then add the bell peppers and the sweet potato. Season with the paprika, garlic powder, and red pepper flakes and toss gently. Transfer to a bowl.

3. Give the pan another spritz of the cooking spray and place it over medium heat. Add the egg whites, stirring, then add the cheese and cook 1 to 2 minutes, until cheese is melted and eggs are scrambled.

4. Spoon the eggs onto plates with the home fries and season with salt and pepper to taste.

Nutrition Info
Calories: 390
Fat: 1 gram
Carbs: 60 grams
Protein: 36 grams
Fiber: 8 grams

Open-Faced Egg and Bacon Sandwiches

Serves 2

Perhaps the most popular breakfast recipe I've developed to date.

TIP: If you can't find fat-free Cheddar cheese, substitute shredded part-skim mozzarella.

2	strips turkey bacon
	Nonstick cooking spray
10	egg whites, or 1¼ cups liquid egg substitute
	Salt and black pepper
4	slices whole-grain bread
½	cup shredded fat-free Cheddar cheese
1¼	cups sliced ripe plum tomatoes

1. Microwave the turkey bacon strips on high power for 3 to 4 minutes, until crispy.
2. Coat a medium nonstick pan with cooking spray and place it over medium heat. Add the egg whites and season with salt and pepper. Cook, stirring frequently, 1½ minutes, until the eggs are scrambled.
3. Toast the bread.
4. Spoon the scrambled eggs on top of each piece of toast. Top each with some of the cheese, turkey bacon, and tomatoes.

Nutrition Info
Calories: 412
Fat: 6 grams
Carbs: 56 grams
Protein: 36 grams
Fiber: 8 grams

SANDWICHES

The components of the sandwiches are completely interchangeable—that is, the caramelized onions of the Roast Beef and Caramelized Onion Wrap (page 237) would be great with the sliced chicken in the Tzatziki Chicken Flatbread (page 241) or the sliced turkey in the Curried Turkey and Pear Sandwich (page 240). And the sauce in the Tzatziki Chicken Flatbread would also be delicious with the turkey or roast beef, and so on. As long as you have the basic sauces and fillings on hand, you can mix and match as you like. Since the first edition of *The Body Reset Diet* came out, I've become a huge fan of the quesadilla (see page 235), which, if you swap the bread for a tortilla, is essentially a grilled cheese sandwich. I've included several quesadilla variations that will keep you and the kids (if you have 'em) full, happy, and healthy.

Chickpea "Tuna" Salad Sandwich

Serves 3 to 4

You don't have to be vegetarian or vegan to enjoy a meat-free meal now and again. The spread can be made in a food processor or by hand.

TIP: Chickpeas are a flavorful, versatile source of protein that have a lot to offer beyond hummus.

1   (14-ounce) can chickpeas, drained and rinsed

1   celery rib, minced

¼   red onion (or 1 small shallot), minced

¼   cup plain fat-free Greek yogurt

1   heaping teaspoon yellow mustard

    Juice of ½ lemon

¾   teaspoon lemon pepper

    Salt

6   to 8 slices sandwich bread

    Mustard, lettuce, and tomato slices, as desired

1. In a food processor, pulse together the chickpeas, celery, and onion until crumbly. (Alternatively, mash the chickpeas, celery, and onion in a bowl with a fork or potato masher.) Add the yogurt, mustard, lemon juice, lemon pepper, and a pinch of salt, and pulse until mostly creamy and only a little chunky. Season to taste with salt.

2. Toast the bread, if desired. Spread a little mustard on each piece of toast. Top half the pieces with some lettuce, followed by some of the sandwich filling. Add a tomato slice and an additional leaf of lettuce (to keep tomato from making the bread soggy), then top with the second piece of bread to each sandwich, and serve.

Nutrition Info

Calories: 281
Fat: 4 grams
Carbs: 55 grams
Protein: 11 grams
Fiber: 6 grams

Quesadilla Master Recipe

Serves 1

Quesadillas are a great way to get your veggies and protein in one tasty bundle. Mix and match your ingredients for different tastes.

TIP: If you don't feel like hand-chopping the veggies, make your filling in the food processor by pulsing the protein and veggies until finely chopped, then adding the cheese and seasoning. You can also buy finely chopped frozen veggies at your grocery store—things like riced cauliflower or broccoli work great!

¼   cup shredded cheese

2 to 3 ounces shredded or finely diced cooked protein

¼   cup finely diced veggies

        Seasonings

        Nonstick cooking spray

1   (12-inch) large tortilla

        Fresh salsa

        Plain fat-free Greek yogurt

1. In a small bowl, stir together the cheese, protein, veggies, and seasonings.

2. Lightly coat a large nonstick skillet with cooking spray and place over medium heat. Put the tortilla in the skillet and immediately cover half of it with your filling.

3. Fold the tortilla in half and press down with a spatula as it cooks for 1 to 2 minutes, allowing the cheese to "bind" the halves together. Cook an additional minute if necessary, until the tortilla is golden brown and toasty, and the cheese is melted.

4. Serve with salsa and Greek yogurt.

Nutrition Info

Calories: 392
Fat: 17 grams
Carbs: 24 grams
Protein: 35 grams
Fiber: 2 grams

Type	Protein	Veggie	Cheese	Seasoning
Classic Chicken	Shredded chicken	2 tablespoons minced bell pepper, 2 tablespoons minced onion	Monterey jack	¼ teaspoon chili powder
Cilantro Lime	Shredded chicken or minced shrimp	2 tablespoons minced fresh cilantro, 2 tablespoons minced fresh spinach	Monterey jack + mozzarella	Zest of 1 lime
Broccoli Cheddar	Diced tofu or chicken	¼ cup finely minced broccoli	Cheddar + mozzarella	Smoked paprika
Pizzadilla	Crumbled Italian-flavored turkey sausage	1 tablespoon tomato sauce, 3 tablespoons minced red and green pepper	Mozzarella + parmesan	¼ teaspoon each dried oregano and basil, onion powder, and garlic powder
Black Bean	Lightly crushed canned black beans	2 tablespoons minced fresh cilantro, 2 tablespoons minced bell peppers	Monterey jack + mozzarella	1 teaspoon minced chipotle chile in adobo sauce
Green Chili Chicken	Shredded cooked chicken	2 tablespoons minced green bell pepper, 2 tablespoons minced fresh cilantro	Monterey jack + mozzarella	2 tablespoons green chile salsa (salsa verde)

Roast Beef and Caramelized Onion Wrap

Serves 1

Roast beef, creamy horseradish, onion, and watercress are a classic sandwich combination.

TIP: Because so little oil is used here, it's important to keep stirring the onion as it cooks—you want it to be soft and golden.

> Nonstick cooking spray
>
> 1   small onion, thinly sliced
>
> 1   whole wheat flatbread
>
> 1   teaspoon prepared horseradish
>
> 1   tablespoon reduced-fat mayonnaise
>
> 3   ounces sliced roast beef
>
> 1   cup coarsely chopped watercress

1. Coat a small nonstick skillet with cooking spray and place it over medium-low heat. Add the onion, reduce the heat to low, and cook for 8 minutes, stirring frequently, until the onion is golden.

2. In a toaster oven or oven preheated to 350°F, warm the flatbread.

3. In a small cup, combine the horseradish and mayonnaise.

4. Spread the horseradish mixture on the warm flatbread. Top with the roast beef, onion, and watercress. Roll up to make a wrap.

Nutrition Info
Calories: 305
Fat: 7 grams
Carbs: 38 grams
Protein: 27 grams
Fiber: 9 grams

Lemon Ricotta Edamame Crostini

Serves 1

This pretty combination makes a perfect lunch on a warm day. It also works well as an elegant appetizer for your next cocktail party.

TIP: Don't skip the lemon peel—it adds a blast of lemon flavor.

- ⅓ cup frozen edamame, thawed
- ½ cup part-skim ricotta
- ½ teaspoon grated lemon peel
- ½ teaspoon fresh lemon juice
- Chopped fresh parsley
- Salt and black pepper
- 2 slices double-fiber whole wheat bread
- ½ cup baby arugula

1. In a small saucepan, cook the edamame according to package directions.
2. In a small bowl, combine the ricotta, lemon peel, lemon juice, and parsley. Season to taste with salt and pepper.
3. Toast the bread.
4. Slather the bread slices with the ricotta mixture, then mound it with the edamame and arugula.

Nutrition Info

Calories: 285
Fat: 9 grams
Carbs: 37 grams
Protein: 23 grams
Fiber: 15 grams

Southwestern Tuna Tortilla Wrap

Serves 2

Salsa is not just for dipping; it also works well as a sandwich spread. Tailor the spiciness of your sandwich filling by selecting mild or hot varieties of salsa.

TIP: Unlike some of the other sandwich recipes, this one serves 2, so save the second sandwich for lunch tomorrow!

6	tablespoons mild or medium salsa
2	tablespoons reduced-fat mayonnaise
1	tablespoon fresh lime juice
2	tablespoons chopped fresh cilantro
1	(6-ounce) can albacore tuna, packed in water
	Salt and black pepper
	Ground cumin
2	whole wheat tortillas
1	cup shredded romaine lettuce

1. In a medium bowl, combine the salsa, mayonnaise, lime juice, and cilantro. Fold in the tuna and season to taste with the salt, pepper, and cumin.

2. Mound the tuna mixture onto the tortillas. Top with the lettuce. Carefully roll up the tortillas to make 2 wraps.

Nutrition Info
Calories: 240
Fat: 6 grams
Carbs: 25 grams
Protein: 29 grams
Fiber: 14 grams

Curried Turkey and Pear Sandwich

Serves 1

Pears are a fiber-rich snack and a sweet addition to this sandwich.

TIP: Pears out of season? Use an apple instead.

- 2   tablespoons plain fat-free Greek yogurt
-      Salt and black pepper
- ¼   teaspoon curry powder
- 2   slices double-fiber whole-grain bread
- 3   ounces sliced turkey
- 1   ripe pear, unpeeled, thinly sliced
- 1   leaf red leaf or romaine lettuce

1. In a small bowl, whisk together the yogurt, salt and pepper to taste, and curry powder.

2. Spread the curried yogurt on 1 slice of bread. Layer on the turkey, pear, and lettuce, and top with the second slice of bread.

Nutrition Info

Calories: 280
Fat: 3 grams
Carbs: 50 grams
Protein: 20 grams
Fiber: 14 grams

Tzatziki Chicken Flatbread

Serves 1

Tzatziki is a Greek or Turkish cucumber yogurt sauce. Here it elevates an easy chicken salad sandwich.

TIP: Be sure to check the Nutrition Facts label when selecting a flatbread at the supermarket. Look for a brand with a high fiber content.

1	teaspoon extra-virgin olive oil
2	teaspoons fresh lemon juice
2	tablespoons plain fat-free Greek yogurt
½	small cucumber, halved and very thinly sliced
1	tablespoon chopped fresh dill
	Salt and black pepper
1	small ripe tomato, chopped
3	ounces sliced cooked boneless, skinless chicken breast
1	whole wheat flatbread

1. Make the tzatziki: In a small bowl, whisk together the olive oil, lemon juice, yogurt, cucumber, dill, salt and pepper.

2. Add the tomato and chicken to the tzatziki and stir to coat.

3. In a toaster oven or oven preheated to 350ºF, warm the flatbread.

4. Pile the chicken salad on the flatbread and serve.

Nutrition Info
Calories: 325
Fat: 10 grams
Carbs: 25 grams
Protein: 39 grams
Fiber: 10 grams

Open-Faced Chicken and Caramelized Onion Sandwich

Serves 2

Thin slices of boneless, skinless chicken breast are sometimes called cutlets, and they cook in just minutes. Substitute an already cooked chicken breast, if you like.

TIP: Cooking onion slices over low heat for a long time caramelizes their natural sugars and lends a sweetness to the sandwich topping.

Nonstick cooking spray

1   large onion, halved and very thinly sliced (about 1½ cups)

1   tablespoon balsamic vinegar

Salt and pepper

2   (2½-ounce) boneless, skinless chicken cutlets

1   (8-inch) piece whole-grain baguette, cut in half

1. Coat a large nonstick skillet with cooking spray and place it over medium-low heat. Add the onion and cook for 15 minutes, stirring frequently. If the onion appears to be scorching, add up to 2 tablespoons water and reduce the heat to low. Add the vinegar and salt to taste. Cook, stirring frequently, for 4 minutes longer, until golden. Scrape the onion onto a plate.

2. Coat the same skillet with more cooking spray and place over medium heat. Season the chicken with salt and pepper and cook for 4 minutes, then turn and cook an additional 4 minutes on the other side, until cooked through.

3. Toast the baguette halves.

4. Top each baguette half with a chicken cutlet and half the onion.

Nutrition Info
Calories: 480
Fat: 13 grams
Carbs: 70 grams
Protein: 20 grams
Fiber: 8 grams

Greek Tuna Melt

Serves 2

*The temperate climate of much of Greece means tomatoes
can be eaten during most of the year. They make a perfect
partner for the tuna and salty feta, with pita wedges for
scooping.*

1   (6-ounce) can white albacore tuna packed in water, drained

1   teaspoon olive oil

1   teaspoon red wine vinegar

    Salt and black pepper

1   large ripe tomato, thinly sliced

¼   cup reduced-fat feta cheese, crumbled (about 1 ounce)

1   teaspoon chopped fresh oregano

2   whole-grain pitas, cut into wedges

1. In a small bowl, toss the tuna with the olive oil, vinegar, and salt and
pepper.

2. On a large microwave-safe plate, arrange the tomato slices so that they
are slightly overlapping. Sprinkle the tomato with the tuna mixture and the
feta cheese. Microwave on high power for 2 minutes, or until the cheese
bubbles and the tuna is warmed through.

3. Sprinkle with the oregano. Serve hot with the pita wedges.

Nutrition Info
Calories: 230
Fat: 6 grams
Carbs: 18 grams
Protein: 26 grams
Fiber: 3 grams

Homemade Gyros

Serves 2

Growing up in Toronto, I used to visit our local Greek area for my favorite gyro lunch.

- 1　teaspoon ground paprika
- ½　teaspoon fresh oregano, or ¼ teaspoon dried
  　Salt and black pepper
- ¾　pound boneless pork loin, thinly sliced
- ½　teaspoon white wine vinegar
  　Nonstick cooking spray
- 2　whole-grain pitas
- ¼　cup tzatziki, homemade (see page 241) or store-bought
- ¼　cup thinly sliced red onion
- 1　ripe tomato, thinly sliced

1. In a small bowl, combine the paprika, oregano, salt, and pepper.

2. Lay the pork slices on a sheet of plastic wrap and cover with another piece of plastic wrap. Use a mallet or the bottom of a heavy saucepan to pound the pork slices to less than ¼ inch thick. Lay the pork slices in a non-reactive 13 by 9–inch dish. Sprinkle with the paprika mixture, then drizzle with the vinegar. Refrigerate for 30 minutes.

3. Preheat the oven to 300°F.

4. Coat a large nonstick skillet with cooking spray and place it over high heat. Add the pork and sauté for 3 minutes, then turn and sauté an additional 3 minutes, until browned and cooked through.

5. Wrap the pitas in foil and warm them in the oven for 15 minutes.

6. Place the pitas on a work surface and layer on the pork, the tzatziki, onion, and tomato slices on top.

Nutrition Info
Calories: 370
Fat: 15 grams
Carbs: 21 grams
Protein: 39 grams
Fiber: 3 grams

SOUPS

Almost-Classic 10-Minute Gazpacho <small>Serves 2</small>

This recipe makes enough for two servings; save the leftovers in a jar in the fridge for up to two days.

TIP: The smoked paprika really takes this gazpacho up a notch! Its rich taste makes it seem like it took a lot longer than 10 minutes to make. For extra spice, add a squirt of hot sauce to your bowl just before eating.

2 to 3 large ripe tomatoes, quartered (about 1 pound)

½   cucumber, peeled and chopped into quarters

½   red bell pepper, cored, seeded, and chopped

½   red onion, roughly chopped

1   garlic clove

½   cup whole or slivered almonds (optional)

2   tablespoons red wine vinegar

1 to 3 cups no-salt/no-sugar-added tomato juice (or vegetable broth or water + bouillon cube)

1   teaspoon smoked paprika

      Salt

2   (3-ounce) servings prepared protein (chopped chicken, shrimp, tofu, or hard-boiled egg; see page 190)

1. In a food processor, pulse the tomatoes, cucumber, bell pepper, onion, garlic, and almonds (if using) until the consistency of a salsa.
2. Add the vinegar, 1 cup of the tomato juice, and the paprika. Blend until smooth and light, adding more liquid until you've reached a smooth, spoonable consistency.
3. Taste and adjust the seasoning, then serve sprinkled with the protein.

Nutrition Info

Calories: 394
Fat: 17 grams
Carbs: 25 grams
Protein: 38 grams
Fiber: 8 grams

Curried Cauliflower Soup

*Place the cauliflower and onion in the oven to roast when
you get home from work, and by the time you've settled in,
they will be ready to toss into the food processor.*

TIP: If you've got a high-speed blender, it will keep the soup
warm as it spins, but you may have to do the blending in two
batches. Better yet, use a food processor and simply reheat
the soup in the microwave or on the stovetop before serving.

	Nonstick cooking spray
2	tablespoons extra-virgin olive oil
1	garlic clove, chopped
1	tablespoon curry powder
½	teaspoon ground cumin
2	cups small cauliflower florets
½	medium onion, diced
3	cups vegetable or chicken broth (or water + 1 bouillon cube)
1	(15-ounce) can low-sodium diced tomatoes
	Salt
¼	cup minced fresh cilantro or mint
4	(3-ounce) servings prepared protein of choice (chicken, shrimp, or tofu; see page 190)

1. Preheat the oven to 375ºF. Coat a baking sheet with nonstick cooking spray.
2. In a large bowl, combine the olive oil, garlic, curry powder, and cumin. Add the cauliflower and onion, and toss until cauliflower is well coated with the spice mixture.
3. Spread the mixture on the baking sheet and roast for 20 to 25 minutes, until the cauliflower is tender.
4. Transfer the roasted veggies to a food processor or high-speed blender. Add the broth and tomatoes, and process until smooth. Taste, and adjust the seasoning as needed.
5. Serve sprinkled with the herbs and offer the protein on the side.

Nutrition Info
Calories: 263
Fat: 11 grams
Carbs: 11 grams
Protein: 31 grams
Fiber: 3 grams

Black Bean Soup with Lime

Serves 4

Rich in fiber and protein, black beans are a powerhouse food. Combining them with lime, garlic, and cumin makes them as delicious as they are nutritious.

TIP: Your whole family will love this hearty soup. It's also a perfect S-meal to make for a small gathering. So, you might not have any leftovers at all. But if you do, store in an airtight container in the fridge; the soup will keep up to four days.

2   tablespoons olive oil

1   red onion, minced

2   garlic cloves, minced

     Zest and juice of 2 limes

½   teaspoon ground cumin

     Salt

2   (15-ounce) cans low-sodium black beans, drained

3   cups chicken or vegetable broth (or water + bouillon cube)

½   cup plain fat-free Greek yogurt

½   cup fresh cilantro, minced

1. Place the olive oil in a soup pot and set over medium heat. When hot, add three-fourths of the onion and all the garlic and cook for 3 to 4 minutes, stirring occasionally, until the onion and garlic are tender.

2. Add the lime zest, cumin, and ½ teaspoon salt, and sauté another minute, until very fragrant.

3. Add the beans and broth, cover, and simmer for 15 minutes, until heated through and the flavors meld.

4. Check the consistency of the soup. If you prefer a smoother, creamier soup, transfer the mixture to a food processor and blend until smooth.

5. Just before serving, add the lime juice and check the seasoning. Sprinkle on the remaining chopped raw onion, and serve with a spoonful of yogurt and a scattering of the cilantro.

Nutrition Info
Calories: 240
Fat: 9 grams
Carbs: 28 grams
Protein: 14 grams
Fiber: 9 grams

Creamy Black Bean and Pumpkin Soup

Serves 2

The flavors of this soup are so rich you'd never guess that the beans and pumpkin come from a can!

TIP: This soup will keep for several days in the refrigerator. You may need to add some liquid when you reheat it.

2 cups canned black beans, rinsed and drained

½ (15-ounce) can pumpkin puree

½ cup chopped canned or fresh tomatoes

Nonstick cooking spray

½ cup chopped onion

Salt and black pepper

Ground cumin

1 (14.5-ounce) can reduced-sodium chicken broth

1 tablespoon sherry vinegar or red wine vinegar

1 tablespoon pumpkin seeds, for garnish

1. In a blender, puree the beans, pumpkin, and tomatoes.

2. Coat a medium saucepan with cooking spray and place it over medium heat. Add the onion and cook for 4 minutes, stirring frequently, until softened. Season with the salt, pepper, and cumin.

3. Add the bean puree and the broth to the pan. Bring to a simmer over medium heat and cook for 20 minutes, stirring occasionally. The soup will be thick.

4. Stir in the vinegar. Garnish with the pumpkin seeds, if desired, and serve.

Nutrition Info
Calories: 390
Fat: 3 grams
Carbs: 67 grams
Protein: 25 grams
Fiber: 16 grams

Sunset Squash Soup

Serves 2

Since this recipe makes 2 servings, save half of it to bring to work for lunch the next day.

TIP: Look for packaged cut squash in the produce section of your grocery store.

　　Nonstick cooking spray
1　small onion, chopped
　　Salt and black pepper
2　cups cubed butternut squash (about ½ squash)
½　(8-ounce) can diced tomatoes
　　Pinch of chopped fresh or dried thyme
2½ cups reduced-sodium chicken broth
1½ cups canned white beans, rinsed and drained
2　cups baby spinach
2　tablespoons grated Parmesan cheese, for garnish

1. Coat a large saucepan with cooking spray and place it over medium-low heat. Add the onion and season with the salt and pepper. Cook for 4 minutes, stirring frequently, until softened.

2. Add the squash, tomatoes, and thyme. Cook for 2 minutes, stirring, to combine the flavors. Add the broth. Increase the heat to high and bring to a simmer. Cook for 15 to 20 minutes, stirring occasionally, until the squash is tender.

3. Add the beans and spinach and cook 3 minutes more, or until warmed through. Garnish the soup with the Parmesan and serve.

Nutrition Info
Calories: 340
Fat: 3 grams
Carbs: 68 grams
Protein: 44 grams
Fiber: 17 grams

Winter's Day Beef with Barley Soup

Barley is traditionally used in beef soups, but feel free to substitute your favorite whole grain.

TIP: Browning the beef adds flavor to the soup, so don't skip this step.

½ cup pearl barley

1½ cups water

   Salt

   Nonstick cooking spray

½ medium onion, chopped

1 cup sliced carrots

   Black pepper

1½ cups sliced button mushrooms

½ cup chopped fresh or canned tomatoes

4 ounces top round steak, sliced

   Minced fresh thyme

3 cups reduced-sodium chicken broth

2 slices double-fiber whole wheat bread

1. In a medium saucepan, combine the barley with the water and a pinch of salt. Bring to a boil over high heat. Reduce the heat to low, cover, and cook for 40 minutes, or until the barley is tender and most of the liquid is absorbed. Fluff with a fork.

2. Coat a large saucepan with cooking spray and place it over medium heat. Add the onion and carrots, season with salt and pepper, and cook for 3 minutes, or until softened. Reduce the heat to low, add the mushrooms and tomatoes, and cook for 6 minutes, stirring frequently, until the mushrooms have released their liquid. Stir in the steak and thyme and cook for 30 seconds more.

3. Add the broth to the pot and bring the soup to a simmer. Cook for 10 minutes to combine the flavors. Stir in the barley and cook until warmed through and thickened.

4. Toast the bread. Serve the toast along with the soup.

Nutrition Info
Calories: 350
Fat: 5 grams
Carbs: 56 grams
Protein: 27 grams
Fiber: 11 grams

Homestyle Chicken Soup

Serves 2

Homemade soup is easy if you are able to pick up a rotisserie chicken at your supermarket. Just make sure to use the meat only, not the skin.

TIP: Serve this soup with some toasted bread to sop up the rich broth.

	Nonstick cooking spray
1	cup chopped carrots
½	cup chopped onion
4	cups reduced-sodium chicken broth
1¼	cups cooked brown rice
1	cup chopped cooked chicken breast
½	cup frozen green peas, thawed
1	slice double-fiber whole wheat bread
2	tablespoons chopped fresh dill, for garnish

1. Coat a large saucepan with cooking spray and place it over medium heat. Cook the carrots and onion for 5 minutes, stirring frequently, until softened. Add the broth, increase the heat to high, and bring to a simmer. Cook for 15 minutes to blend the flavors and cook the carrots.
2. Stir in the rice, chicken, and peas. Heat until warmed through.
3. Toast the bread.
4. Garnish servings of the soup with the dill. Cut the toast in half and serve it alongside the soup.

Nutrition Info
Calories: 335
Fat: 4 grams
Carbs: 46 grams
Protein: 26 grams
Fiber: 8 grams

Golden Split Pea Soup Serves 2

Pea soup is incredibly high in protein and fiber. It tastes
hearty but is still light on your waistline.

½   teaspoon olive oil

2   carrots, chopped

1   small onion, chopped

1   celery rib, chopped

    Salt and black pepper

1   cup dried green or yellow split peas

½   ham hock, well rinsed

1   teaspoon minced fresh thyme

3   cups reduced-sodium chicken or vegetable broth

2   slices rye or whole-grain bread

1. In a large saucepan over medium-low heat, warm the olive oil. Add the carrots, onion, and celery. Season with salt and pepper and cook for 4 minutes, stirring frequently. Add the split peas, ham hock, thyme, and broth. Bring to a simmer, then reduce the heat and cook for 40 minutes, stirring frequently. If the soup is looking dry, add up to 1 cup of water to maintain a soupy consistency.
2. Using a 1-cup measure or a ladle, transfer about half the soup to a blender or food processor. Puree until smooth. (Alternatively, puree the soup in the pot with an immersion blender.)
3. Remove the ham hock from the pot and chop about ¼ cup meat from the bone, then return the ham to the soup. (Discard the bone.) Return the pureed soup to the pot, stir well, and warm through.
4. Toast the bread and cut it into triangles. Season the soup with additional salt and pepper, and serve with the toast triangles alongside.

Nutrition Info
Calories: 370
Fat: 11g grams
Carbs: 25 grams
Protein: 44 grams
Fiber: 12 grams

SALADS

NOTE: Many of these recipes make enough for two salads—if you're not going to eat it all right away, dress only half of it and store the remaining dressing and salad ingredients separately so they don't get soggy. (I like to use glass jars so I can grab them and go.)

Shaved Sprouts Salad

Serves 2

You may think you don't like Brussels sprouts, but you probably haven't tried them raw. With the green of the sprouts and the purple of the pomegranate seeds and red onion, this salad looks as good as it tastes.

TIP: Look for bagged shaved Brussels sprouts in the produce section of your grocery store. If not available, buy shredded green cabbage, or trim the hard stem ends from whole Brussels sprouts, then shred them with a box grater or in a food processor fitted with the shredding disk.

For the dressing:

½ ripe avocado

3 tablespoons lemon juice, red wine vinegar, or a combination

1 teaspoon Dijon mustard

½ teaspoon sea salt

2 tablespoons minced fresh herbs (optional; parsley, dill, mint, and cilantro work well)

For the salad:

3   **cups Brussels sprouts shavings**

¼   **medium red onion, thinly sliced**

1   **cup pomegranate seeds**

1   **cup chopped cooked chicken breast**

2   **tablespoons shredded Parmesan cheese (optional)**

1. In a blender, combine the avocado, lemon juice, mustard, salt, and herbs. Blend until creamy. The dressing should be a thick but pourable consistency; if too thick, add a little water a teaspoon at a time until desired consistency.

2. In a large bowl, toss together the sprouts and red onion. Carefully fold in the pomegranate seeds, chicken, and then the dressing. Serve sprinkled with cheese, if you'd like.

Nutrition Info
Calories: 307
Fat: 14 grams
Carbs: 32 grams
Protein: 20 grams
Fiber: 9 grams

Chopped Greek Salad

Serves 2

This is a great salad for a hot day, especially if your peppers and cucumbers are chilled. The juicy crunch of the vegetables will help you stay hydrated, as well.

TIP: As an alternative, serve this over a bed of chopped romaine for a more traditional salad.

For the dressing:

2   ripe medium tomatoes, diced

    Salt

2   tablespoons olive oil

3   tablespoons red wine vinegar

1   teaspoon dried oregano, or 1 tablespoon minced fresh

For the salad:

2   bell peppers, cored, seeded, and chopped

2   English cucumbers, peeled and diced

1   red onion, diced

¼   cup chopped pitted Kalamata olives

¼   cup crumbled reduced-fat feta cheese

1   cup chopped cooked shrimp or chicken

1. In a large bowl, combine the tomatoes and salt. Let sit about 10 minutes to draw out the liquid.
2. Place the olive oil, vinegar, and oregano in a container with a tight-fitting lid. Shake to combine well. Drain the liquid from the tomatoes into the dressing, cover, and shake again.
3. In a medium bowl, toss together the bell peppers, cucumbers, red onion, and olives. Add the cheese, shrimp or chicken, and dressing and toss gently to mix until ingredients are well dressed. Serve at once.

Nutrition Info
Calories: 386
Fat: 19 grams
Carbs: 32 grams
Protein: 26 grams
Fiber: 7 grams

Sesame Red and Green Slaw

Serves 3 to 4

Red cabbage is a great thing to eat more of, as it has more antioxidants than its green counterpart. Here, it is paired with broccoli "slaw" for an interesting blend.

TIP: If you don't have or can't find tahini, use almond or peanut butter instead. Broccoli slaw can be found, bagged, in the refrigerated produce section of your grocery.

For the dressing:

- 2　　tablespoons tahini
- 3　　tablespoons toasted sesame oil
- ¼　　cup lemon juice, rice wine vinegar, or a combination
- ⅓　　cup plain fat-free Greek yogurt, light mayonnaise, or a combination

For the salad:

- ½　　medium red cabbage, shredded (about 4 cups)
- ½　　medium red onion, thinly sliced
- 2　　cups broccoli slaw
- 2　　cups shredded cooked chicken
- ½　　cup whole almonds, chopped
- 　　Salt

1. In a small bowl, whisk together the tahini, sesame oil, lemon juice, and yogurt to make a smooth, creamy dressing.
2. In a large bowl, toss together the red cabbage, red onion, broccoli, chicken, and almonds. Fold in the dressing, stirring until the ingredients are lightly coated. Season to taste with salt.

Nutrition Info
Calories: 428
Fat: 29 grams
Carbs: 18 grams
Fiber: 6 grams
Protein: 27 grams

Black Bean and Lime-Mango Salad   Serves 1

For added flavor and color, serve this colorful salad on a bed of chopped lettuce or baby arugula.

TIP: Use fresh mango if it's in season; otherwise, substitute thawed frozen chopped mango.

1	teaspoon grated lime zest
3	tablespoons fresh lime juice
1	teaspoon extra-virgin olive oil
1	cup canned black beans, rinsed and drained
½	cup chopped peeled cucumber
½	cup chopped fresh mango
¼	cup chopped avocado
	Salt and black pepper
	Ground cumin

In a medium bowl, whisk together the lime zest, lime juice, and olive oil until well blended. Add the beans, cucumber, mango, and avocado and toss to coat well. Season to taste with salt and pepper, and sprinkle on the cumin.

Nutrition Info
Calories: 390
Fat: 10 grams
Carbs: 59 grams
Protein: 19 grams
Fiber: 22 grams

Grilled Steak and Baby Spinach Salad

Serves 1

This is a healthier version of a fancy bistro salad—bursting with texture and flavor. Make it tonight!

TIP: If possible, use an intensely flavored extra-virgin olive oil for your salad dressings. The less expensive olive oils are best for cooked dishes.

1	(2-ounce) piece boneless top round steak
	Salt and black pepper
2	teaspoons balsamic vinegar
1	teaspoon extra-virgin olive oil
2	cups baby spinach leaves
½	fennel bulb, trimmed and thinly sliced
½	cup seedless red grapes, cut into halves
10	whole almonds, chopped
1	whole wheat flatbread

1. Preheat a grill to very hot or heat a grill pan over high heat. Season the steak to taste with the salt and pepper. Grill the steak for 5 minutes on each side, or until a thermometer inserted in the center registers 145°F for medium-rare, 160°F for medium, or 165°F for well-done, as desired. Let stand 10 minutes, then thinly slice.

2. In a medium bowl, whisk the vinegar and olive oil until well blended.

3. Add the spinach, fennel, and grapes, tossing to coat well. Add the steak slices to the bowl and toss again. Garnish with the almonds, and serve with the flatbread.

Nutrition Info
Calories: 355
Fat: 11 grams
Carbs: 37 grams
Protein: 32 grams
Fiber: 13 grams

Dijon Lentil Salad with Baby Spinach   Serves 1

This is one of those magical dishes that can be served warm, at room temperature, or chilled, making it a great bring-to-work lunch option.

TIP: The cooking time for the lentils will vary depending on the type of lentil used. If you can find the tiny le Puy lentils, they will cook in 20 minutes; larger types will take closer to 25 minutes.

	Nonstick cooking spray
2	tablespoons finely chopped shallot or onion
½	cup lentils
2	cups water
1	teaspoon extra-virgin olive oil
2	teaspoons Dijon mustard
2	teaspoons red wine vinegar
	Salt and black pepper
1	cup baby spinach

1. Coat a medium saucepan with cooking spray and place it over medium heat. Add the shallot and sauté for 2 minutes, stirring, until lightly browned. Add the lentils and water, and bring to a simmer. Lower the heat and cook for 20 to 25 minutes, adding more water if needed, until lentils are just tender. Drain, if needed.

2. In a medium bowl, whisk together the olive oil, mustard, and vinegar. Stir in the warm lentils. Season to taste with salt and pepper.

3. Line a shallow bowl with the spinach. Mound the lentil salad on top and serve.

Nutrition Info
Calories: 300
Fat: 5 grams
Carbs: 42 grams
Protein: 20 grams
Fiber: 17 grams

Chicken and Zucchini Salad with Buttermilk Dressing

Serves 2

Who needs a heavy mayonnaise-based potato salad when you can have something like this?

TIP: For best flavor, slice the zucchini as thin as possible.

3	tablespoons buttermilk
1	tablespoon white wine vinegar
1	tablespoon chopped fresh dill
	Salt and black pepper
1	small zucchini, halved lengthwise and sliced into paper-thin half-moons
1	cup cherry tomatoes, cut into halves
¾	cup chopped cooked chicken
2	cups baby arugula

In a medium bowl, whisk together the buttermilk, vinegar, dill, salt, and pepper. Fold in the zucchini, tomatoes, and chicken. Serve on a bed of the arugula.

Nutrition Info
Calories: 320
Fat: 5 grams
Carbs: 31 grams
Protein: 42 grams
Fiber: 9 grams

Lemon Quinoa with Spring Vegetables

Serves 1

Use any combination of spring vegetables: asparagus, green peas, snap peas, scallions. The steaming time is about the same for all of them.

TIP: Some sugar snap peas have a tough string running along the top of the pod. To remove it, snap off the tip and pull down on the string.

2	tablespoons fresh lemon juice
1	garlic clove, minced
1½	cups water
⅓	cup quinoa
1	cup chopped spring vegetables, fresh or frozen
½	cup rinsed and drained canned chickpeas
	Salt and black pepper
¼	cup chopped fresh parsley

1. In a medium bowl, whisk together the lemon juice and garlic.
2. In a small saucepan, bring the water to a boil. Add the quinoa, cover, and cook for 7 minutes. Uncover the pan, place the vegetables in a colander or steamer basket, and set it over the cooking quinoa. Cook an additional 5 minutes, or until the vegetables are crisp-tender and the quinoa is tender.
3. Transfer the vegetables to the bowl with the dressing and toss to coat well.
4. Fold in the warm quinoa and chickpeas, then season to taste with salt and pepper. Garnish with the parsley.

Nutrition Info
Calories: 390
Fat: 6 grams
Carbs: 67 grams
Protein: 20 grams
Fiber: 15 grams

Easy Niçoise Salad   Serves 2

This dish is not only delicious but also truly beautiful, so be sure to plate it thoughtfully.

4	ounces green beans, trimmed and cut in half
1	(6-ounce) can white albacore tuna packed in water, drained
¼	cup red wine vinegar
	Salt
4	cups baby lettuce leaves
1	medium ripe tomato, thinly sliced
2	hard-cooked eggs, split in half and yolks discarded
4	thin slices whole wheat baguette

1. Bring a small saucepan of water to a boil over high heat. Add the beans and cook for 3 minutes or until tender–crisp. Drain and rinse with cool water.

2. In a small bowl, mix the tuna and 2 tablespoons of the vinegar. Season to taste with salt.

3. On a medium platter, arrange the lettuce, tomato slices, beans, and tuna. Drizzle the salad with the remaining 2 tablespoons vinegar. Slice the egg whites and arrange them on top or around the edges. Serve with the baguette slices.

Nutrition Info
Calories: 360
Fat: 8 grams
Carbs: 38 grams
Protein: 33 grams
Fiber: 7 grams

Mexican Chicken Salad with Spicy Salsa Dressing

Serves 2

No stove-top cooking necessary! I love this salad because of the easy prep and the way it tastes.

1   teaspoon fajita seasoning mix

    Pinch of ground cumin

    Salt and black pepper

1   (6-ounce) boneless, skinless chicken breast

1   cup fat-free sour cream

1   cup mild or hot salsa

1   head iceberg lettuce, coarsely chopped

1½ cups canned corn, drained

1. In a medium bowl, combine the seasoning mix, cumin, and salt and pepper. Put the chicken in the bowl and turn to coat it thoroughly.

2. Place the chicken on a microwave-safe plate, cover, and microwave on high power for 6 minutes, until cooked through. Let cool slightly.

3. In a blender, combine the sour cream and salsa. Pulse until the mixture appears dark pink and is smooth; if the dressing is too thick, thin it with a little water.

4. Cut the chicken breast into bite-size pieces. In a large bowl, toss the lettuce, chicken, corn, and dressing to coat well. Serve immediately.

Nutrition Info

Calories: 360

Fat: 4 grams

Carbs: 58 grams

Protein: 35 grams

Fiber: 9 grams

Argentinean Steak Salad with Mustard-Cilantro Vinaigrette

Serves 2

Bison steaks are a great lean alternative to beef. The meat is best served medium-rare. If you can't find bison, look for a sirloin tip side or top round steak, as these are the leanest cuts of beef that also have a good flavor.

1½	teaspoons Dijon mustard
¼	cup white wine vinegar
2	tablespoons dried cilantro leaves
	Salt and black pepper
1	(6-ounce) boneless bison steak
1	teaspoon ground cumin
1	teaspoon ground coriander
	Nonstick cooking spray
4	bunches watercress
5	medium radishes, thinly sliced

1. In a small bowl, whisk together the mustard, vinegar, cilantro, and salt and pepper to taste.
2. Season the meat with the cumin, coriander, and additional salt and pepper.
3. Coat a small nonstick skillet with cooking spray and place over medium-high heat. Sear the meat on both sides for 90 seconds, or until a thermometer inserted in the center registers 145°F for medium-rare, 160°F for medium, or 165°F for well-done, as desired. Let the meat rest for 1 minute, then thinly slice.
4. In a large bowl, toss the watercress with the vinaigrette. Arrange the watercress on a serving plate. Top with the sliced steak and garnish with the radishes.

Nutrition Info
Calories: 433
Fat: 7 grams
Carbs: 64 grams
Protein: 35 grams
Fiber: 10 grams

STIR-FRIES

9-Minute Shrimp and Asparagus Stir-Fry

Serves 4

This is a great thing to serve when friends are coming over—it's delicious, and it means you can stick to the Body Reset Diet (and in only 9 minutes, no less!) even while entertaining.

TIP: The longest part of this recipe is letting the frozen shrimp thaw. If you can, pull the shrimp out of the freezer in the morning, set it into a colander over a bowl, and place it in the fridge to thaw.

2	tablespoons avocado oil
1	small onion, thinly sliced
4	garlic cloves, minced
1	pound peeled frozen shrimp, thawed
1	bunch fresh asparagus, trimmed and chopped into bite–size pieces
	Zest and juice of 1 lemon
	Salt
1½	teaspoons lemon pepper
¼	cup minced fresh parsley

1. Heat the oil in a large skillet over medium-high heat. Add the onion, garlic, and shrimp, and cook 2 to 3 minutes, until the onion is translucent and the garlic is fragrant.

2. Turn the heat to high, then add the asparagus, lemon zest, salt, and lemon pepper and cook an additional 5 to 7 minutes, stirring frequently, until the shrimp are opaque and cooked through and the asparagus is tender.

3. Drizzle with the lemon juice and sprinkle with the parsley just before serving.

Nutrition Info

Calories: 171
Fat: 3 grams
Carbs: 8 grams
Protein: 28 grams
Fiber: 2 grams

Kung Pao-ish Chicken

Serves 4

To make things simpler, I often buy prepared ginger and garlic paste in the refrigerated produce or freezer section of my local market. If you are using these prepared pastes, just use half the amount this recipe calls for, as their flavor is more concentrated.

TIP: The arrowroot powder or cornstarch is optional, but it provides a thicker, more restaurant-style sauce. And if you like things spicy, add a squirt or two of sriracha to the sauce.

- 2 tablespoons toasted sesame oil
- ⅓ cup sodium-reduced soy sauce
- 1 tablespoon arrowroot powder or cornstarch (optional)
- 1 tablespoon honey, maple syrup, or sweetener of choice
- 1 pound boneless, skinless chicken breasts, cut into bite-size pieces
- 2 tablespoons minced fresh ginger
- 2 garlic cloves, minced
- 1 bunch scallions, green and white parts minced
- 2 bell peppers, cored, seeded, and diced
- 2 celery ribs, trimmed and diced
- ¼ cup almonds, peanuts, or cashews, chopped

1. In a jar with a lid, combine 1 tablespoon of the sesame oil with the soy sauce, arrowroot (if using), and honey. Shake to combine.

2. Place the chicken in a zippered plastic bag. Add half the sauce, seal, and squish with your hands to coat the chicken with the seasoning. Let marinate for at least 30 minutes.

3. In a large skillet or wok, heat the remaining tablespoon oil over medium-high heat. Add the ginger, garlic, and scallions, and sauté 1 to 2 minutes, until very fragrant.

4. Open the plastic bag and add the chicken to the skillet. Stir in the bell peppers and celery and continue to cook for 5 to 7 minutes, stirring frequently, until the vegetables and chicken are tender, cooked, and nicely browned on all sides.

5. Reduce the heat to low, add the remaining sauce, and simmer 4 to 6 minutes, until the sauce is thickened. Fold in the nuts just before serving.

Nutrition Info
Calories: 404
Fat: 20 grams
Carbs: 19 grams
Protein: 38 grams
Fiber: 3 grams

10-Minute Stir-Fry

Serves 2

Simple, satisfying, and infinitely adaptable, this meal should become a staple weekend supper.

TIP: Any veggies will work in this anytime stir-fry.

Nonstick cooking spray

7 ounces chicken tenders

2 cups frozen mixed vegetables, thawed

¼ cup reduced-sodium soy sauce

¼ cup reduced-sodium chicken broth

1 tablespoon creamy peanut butter

1 teaspoon cornstarch (optional, but makes for a thicker, more velvety sauce)

1½ cups cooked brown rice, warm

1. Coat a large nonstick skillet with cooking spray and place over medium-high heat. Add the chicken and stir-fry for 4 minutes, until pieces are lightly browned but not cooked through. Add the vegetables and stir-fry for 2 more minutes. Stir in the soy sauce.

2. Pour in the broth, then add the peanut butter and sprinkle in the cornstarch, if using. Cook for 2 more minutes, stirring to blend in the peanut butter and combine the flavors. Serve over the rice.

Nutrition Info

Calories: 565
Fat: 22 grams
Carbs: 65 grams
Protein: 23 grams
Fiber: 5 grams

Creamy Spinach and Chickpea Stir-Fry

Serves 1

This is our easy adaptation of sag paneer, a classic Indian dish. And remember, the spinach will look like a lot when you first put it in the skillet, but it will definitely cook down.

TIP: Buttermilk lends the creamy texture here—the recipe won't work as well with fat-free milk.

Nonstick cooking spray

½ cup canned chickpeas, rinsed and drained

2 garlic cloves, minced

½ teaspoon ground cumin

8 ounces baby spinach, coarsely chopped

½ cup buttermilk

Salt and black pepper

2 tablespoons crumbled reduced-fat feta cheese

1. Coat a large nonstick skillet with cooking spray and place over medium-low heat. Add the chickpeas, garlic, and cumin and cook for 30 seconds, stirring. Add the spinach, cover, and let sit for 30 seconds. Uncover and stir-fry for 2 minutes, or until the spinach is wilted.

2. Stir in the buttermilk and cook until the liquid evaporates. Season to taste with salt and pepper. Sprinkle on the feta just before serving.

Nutrition Info
Calories: 320
Fat: 8 grams
Carbs: 46 grams
Protein: 22 grams
Fiber: 11 grams

Tuscan White Bean and Kale Bruschetta Serves 1

To ensure easy low-fat cooking, invest in a good nonstick skillet. You'll use less oil and need less cleanup time.

TIP: Lots of flatbreads are available in supermarkets today— check the Nutrition Facts to compare their fiber contents.

> Nonstick cooking spray
> 1   cup chopped fresh kale
> 2   garlic cloves, minced
> ⅓   cup canned cannellini beans, rinsed and drained
> 1   tablespoon water
> 1   teaspoon fresh lemon juice
>   Salt and black pepper
> 1   whole wheat flatbread
>   Snipped fresh chives

1. Coat a medium nonstick skillet with cooking spray and set it over medium heat. Add the kale and stir-fry for 3 minutes, until wilted. Add the garlic and stir-fry for 30 more seconds. Add the beans and water, reduce the heat to low, and cook for 1 minute, until warmed through. Stir in the lemon juice and salt and pepper to taste.

2. Toast the flatbread. Spoon the warm kale mixture onto the flatbread, then sprinkle with the chives.

Nutrition Info
Calories: 310
Fat: 6 grams
Carbs: 50 grams
Protein: 22 grams
Fiber: 15 grams

Coconut Chicken Curry

Serves 2

A quick toasting of the spices brings out the exotic flavors in this super-quick curry dish.

TIP: Since everything cooks so quickly, it's a good idea to have all the stir-fry ingredients prepped before you start cooking.

	Nonstick cooking spray
1	tablespoon curry powder
½	teaspoon ground cumin
7	ounces chicken tenders
1	large apple, unpeeled, cored, and cut into chunks
1	cup reduced-sodium chicken broth
½	cup light coconut milk
2	cups cooked barley or brown rice, warm

1. Coat a large nonstick saucepan with cooking spray and place it over medium heat. Add the curry powder and cumin and stir-fry for 10 seconds. Add the chicken and apple and stir-fry for 1 minute more, or until they are browned and coated with the spices.

2. Add the broth and coconut milk and simmer for 10 minutes, stirring occasionally, until the chicken is cooked through and the sauce has thickened. Serve over the barley or brown rice.

Nutrition Info
Calories: 400
Fat: 7 grams
Carbs: 60 grams
Protein: 27 grams
Fiber: 9 grams

Ginger Shrimp with Chard and Bell Peppers

Serves 2

*Feel free to substitute another leafy green for the chard—
spinach, kale, or broccoli rabe are all good options. Note
that the cooking time will vary depending on the green used.*

TIP: Toasted sesame oil is darker and richer than conventional
sesame oil. You need only a small amount for a big flavor boost.

2	teaspoons reduced-sodium soy sauce
2	teaspoons rice wine vinegar
1	teaspoon toasted sesame oil
	Nonstick cooking spray
1	red bell pepper, cored, seeded, and thinly sliced
8	ounces fresh chard, trimmed and thinly sliced
2	teaspoons finely chopped peeled fresh ginger
3	tablespoons water
6	ounces frozen cooked shrimp, thawed
1½	cups cooked brown rice, warm

1. In a small bowl, whisk together the soy sauce, vinegar, and sesame oil.

2. Coat a medium nonstick skillet with cooking spray and place it over medium heat. Add the bell pepper and stir-fry for 2 minutes. Add the chard, ginger, and water and stir-fry for 4 more minutes, until the chard is wilted.

3. Add the shrimp, stir quickly, and drizzle in the sauce. Stir-fry for 2 more minutes, until the pepper and chard are crisp-tender and the shrimp is warmed through. Serve over the rice.

Nutrition Info
Calories: 355
Fat: 8 grams
Carbs: 47 grams
Protein 26 grams
Fiber: 7 grams

Shrimp and Noodle Stir-Fry

Serves 2

Frozen shrimp is a must-have for quick meals; not only are the shrimp already shelled and deveined but they are usually cooked as well. Wear kitchen gloves when handling the chiles.

2   ounces soba or udon noodles
      Nonstick cooking spray
½   fresh red chile, chopped
2   garlic cloves, minced
3   ounces frozen medium shelled and deveined cooked shrimp, thawed (about 8 or 9 shrimp)
1   baby bok choy or 4 ounces fresh spinach, shredded
2   tablespoons frozen green peas, thawed
1   tablespoon reduced-sodium soy sauce
1   tablespoon sweet chile sauce

1. Cook the noodles according to package directions, then drain.
2. Coat a large nonstick skillet with cooking spray and place it over medium-high heat. Add the chile and garlic and sauté for 1 minute, stirring frequently.
3. Add the shrimp, bok choy, and peas and cook for 3 minutes longer, stirring frequently. Add the cooked noodles, soy sauce, and chile sauce, stir to blend, and heat until warmed through.

Nutrition Info
Calories: 407
Fat: 5 grams
Carbs: 46 grams
Protein: 35 grams
Fiber: 6 grams

Spicy Beef Stir-Fry   Serves 2

Chinese black bean sauce is a salty-bitter blend of fermented black beans and garlic. It is available in the Asian foods sections of most supermarkets.

1	(8-ounce) piece flank steak, cut into 1-inch cubes
3	tablespoons reduced-sodium soy sauce
3	tablespoons fresh orange juice
2	tablespoons black bean sauce
1	tablespoon sweet chile paste
	Nonstick cooking spray
¼	broccoli head, stem thinly sliced and florets cut into small pieces
¼	cup water
4	ounces bean sprouts
1½	cups cooked brown rice, warm
	Scallion green, sliced

1. In a medium bowl, combine the beef cubes with 2 tablespoons of the soy sauce and let sit for at least 30 minutes.

2. In a small bowl, whisk together the remaining tablespoon soy sauce, the orange juice, black bean sauce, and chile paste.

3. Coat a large nonstick skillet with cooking spray and set it over medium-high heat. Add the broccoli and cook for 2 minutes, stirring frequently. Add the water, cover, and cook for 1 minute more, until the broccoli stem pieces are tender-crisp. Transfer the broccoli to a platter.

4. Lightly coat the skillet with more cooking spray and place it over medium heat. Add the meat and cook for 2 minutes, stirring constantly. Pour in the sauce, stir, then add the broccoli and the bean sprouts. Cook for 1 minute, or until everything is warmed through. Serve over the rice and garnish with the scallion green.

Nutrition Info

Calories: 470
Fat: 16 grams
Carbs: 38 grams
Protein: 45 grams
Fiber: 4 grams

Shrimp and Rice Stir-Fry

Serves 2

If you think Chinese food is unhealthy, think again! This healthy at-home stir-fry beats any takeout, in terms of flavor and goodness.

1	pound shrimp, peeled and deveined
	Nonstick cooking spray
1½	cups cooked brown rice
1½	teaspoons garlic powder
2	cups broccoli florets
¼	cup slivered scallions, green and white parts
2	teaspoons sesame seeds
¼	cup reduced-sodium soy sauce

1. Remove the tails from the shrimp and cut the shrimp into bite-size pieces.

2. Coat a large nonstick skillet with cooking spray and place it over medium-high heat. Add the shrimp and cook, stirring frequently, for 2 minutes, until nearly cooked. Transfer to a plate.

3. Coat the same skillet with a little more cooking spray. Add the rice and garlic powder and cook for 1 minute, stirring constantly so the rice does not burn. Add the broccoli, continuing to stir; when the broccoli turns bright green, in about 1 minute, add the shrimp, scallions, sesame seeds, and soy sauce. Cook for 1 minute longer, then serve.

Nutrition Info
Calories: 407
Fat: 5 grams
Carbs: 44 grams
Protein: 46 grams
Fiber: 6 grams

Acknowledgments

My family for everything that matters.

My literary agent, Andy Barzvi, who believed in me first, then made sure everyone else did, too.

Wendy Heller for being half lawyer and half sister.

Laura Moser for helping me find the words . . . then putting them in the right order.

Susan Ott for the delicious recipes.

Kate Hanley for helping me reimagine and update.

Danielle Curtis and Ursula Cary for making this book become a reality.

My amazing clients for their loyalty and focus.

Endnotes

INTRODUCTION

1 P. G. Turner and C. E. Lefevre, "Instagram Use Is Linked to Increased Symptoms of Orthorexia Nervosa," *Eating and Weight Disorders* 22, no. 2 (2017): 277–284, doi: 10.1007/s40519-017-0364-2.

2 S. Bo et al., "University Courses, Eating Problems and Muscle Dysmorphia: Are There Any Associations?," *Journal of Translational Medicine* 12 (2014): 221, doi: 10.1186/s12967-014-0221-2.

3 U.S. Department of Health and Human Services Center for Disease Control and Prevention, "National Diabetes Statistics Report 2020: Estimate of Diabetes and Its Burden in the United States," https://www.cdc.gov/diabetes/pdfs/data/statistics/national-diabetes-statistics-report.pdf.

CHAPTER 1

1 International Food Information Council Foundation, "2012 Food & Health Survey," https://foodinsight.org/2012-food-and-health-survey.

2 International Food Information Council Foundation, "2018 Food & Health Survey," https://foodinsight.org/wp-content/uploads/2018/05/2018 -FHS-Report-FINAL.pdf.

3 Melinda M. Manore, "Dietary Supplements for Improving Body Composition and Reducing Body Weight: Where Is the Evidence?," *International Journal of Sport Nutrition and Exercise Metabolism* 22, no. 2 (2012): 139–154, doi: 10.1123/ijsnem.22.2.139.

4 "Body Building, Diet Supplements Linked to Liver Damage: Study," *HealthDay News,* May 22, 2012, https://www.medicinenet.com/script/main/ art.asp?articlekey=158468.

5 "FDA Requests the Withdrawal of the Weight-Loss Drug Belviq, Belviq XYR (lorcaserin) from the Market," FDA Drug Safety Communication, February 13, 2020, https://www.fda.gov/drugs/drug-safety-and-availability/ fda-requests-withdrawal-weight-loss-drug-belviq-belviq-xr-lorcaserin -market.

6 KBV Research, "Global Meal Replacement Products Market (2019–2025)," November 2019, https://www.reportlinker.com/p05832291/Global-Meal -Replacement-Products-Market.html?utm_source=PRN.

7 "Leading Health and Fitness Apps in the U.S. 2018, by Users," Statista .com, November 20, 2019, https://www.statista.com/statistics/650748/health -fitness-app-usage-usa.

8 Stephanie Powers, "7 Popular Diet Plans and What They Cost," *Investopedia,* updated March 6, 2020, https://www.investopedia.com/financial-edge/ 0211/7-popular-diet-plans-and-what-they-cost.aspx.

9 Tanza Loudenback and Liz Knueven, "What Average Americans Spend on Groceries Every Month in 22 Major Cities," *Business Insider,* March 5,

2020, https://www.businessinsider.com/personal-finance/what-americans
-spend-on-groceries-every-month-2019-4.

10 FAQs, https://www.jennycraig.com/faqs#jc-cost, accessed March 23, 2020.

11 John F. Trepanowski et al., "Effect of Alternate-Day Fasting on Weight
Loss, Weight Maintenance, and Cardioprotection among Metabolically
Healthy Obese Adults: A Randomized Clinical Trial," *JAMA Internal Medicine* 177, no. 7 (2017): 930–938, doi: 10.1001/jamainternmed.2017.0936.

12 Ma Xiumei et al., "Skipping Breakfast Is Associated with Overweight
and Obesity: A Systematic Review and Meta-analysis," *Obesity Research & Clinical Practice* 14, no. 1 (2020): 1–8, doi: 10.1016/j.orcp.2019.12.002.

13 Sonia Gómez-Martínez et al., "Eating Habits and Total and Abdominal Fat in Spanish Adolescents: Influence of Physical Activity. The AVENA
Study," *Journal of Adolescent Health* 50, no. 4 (2011): 403–409, doi: 10.1016/
j.jadohealth.2011.08.016.

14 Traci Mann et al., "Medicare's Search for Effective Obesity Treatments:
Diets Are Not the Answer," *American Psychologist* 62, no. 3 (2007): 220–233,
doi: 10.1037/0003-066X.62.3.220.

15 Michael R. Lowe et al., "Dieting and Restrained Eating as Prospective Predictors of Weight Gain," *Frontiers in Psychology* 4 (2013): 577, doi:
10.3389/fpsyg.2013.00577.

16 Cara B. Ebbeling et al., "Effects of Dietary Composition on Energy Expenditure during Weight-Loss Maintenance," *JAMA* 307, no. 24 (2012):
2627–2634, doi: 10.1001/jama.2012.6607.

17 Marlen A. van Baak and Edwin C. M. Mariman, "Dietary Strategies for
Weight Loss Maintenance," *Nutrients* 11, no. 8 (2019): 1916, doi: 10.3390/
nu11081916.

18 Gary Taubes, *Why We Get Fat* (New York: Anchor Books, 2010), 47.

19 Ibid.

20 John Cloud, "Why Exercise Won't Make You Thin," *Time*, August 9,
2009. 12 James H. O'Keefe et al., "Potential adverse cardiovascular effects
from excessive endurance exercise," *Mayo Clinic Proceedings* 87, no. 6 (June
2012), doi: 10.1016/j.mayocp.2012.04.005.

21 Radiological Society of North America, "Male Triathletes May Be Putting Their Heart Health at Risk," November 21, 2017, https://press.rsna.org/timssnet/media/pressreleases/14_pr_target.cfm?id=1981.

22 Maureen Brogan et al., "Freebie Rhabdomyolysis: A Public Health Concern. Spin Class–Induced Rhabdomyolysis," *American Journal of Medicine* 130, no. 4 (2017): 484–487, doi: 10.1016/j.amjmed.2016.11.004.

23 Taija Finni et al., "Inactivity Time Is Independent of Exercise," *Scandinavian Journal of Medicine & Science in Sports* 24 (2014): 211–219, doi: 10.1111/j.1600-0838.2012.01456.x.

24 Kyle Mandsager et al., "Association of Cardiorespiratory Fitness with Long-Term Mortality among Adults Undergoing Exercise Treadmill Testing," *JAMA Network Open* 1, no. 6 (2018): e183605, doi: 10.1001/jamanetworkopen.2018.3605.

CHAPTER 3

1 Kate L. Brookie, Georgia I. Best, and Tamlin S. Connor, "Intake of Raw Fruits and Vegetables Is Associated with Better Mental Health than Intake of Processed Fruits and Vegetables," *Frontiers in Psychology* 9 (2018): 487, doi: 10.3389/fpsyg.2018.00487.

2 Maeve C. Cosgrove et al., "Dietary Nutrient Intakes and Skin-Aging Appearance among Middle-Aged American Women," *American Journal of Clinical Nutrition* 86, no. 4 (2007): 1225–1231, doi: 10.1093/ajcn/86.4.1225.

3 Jon A. Halvorsen et al., "Is the Association between Acne and Mental Distress Influenced by Diet? Results from a Cross-Sectional Population Study among 3775 Late Adolescents in Oslo, Norway," *BMC Public Health* 9 (2009): 340, doi: 10.1186/1471-2458-9-340.

4 Helena Pachón, Rebecca J. Stoltzfus, and Raymond P. Glahn, "Homogenization, Lyophilization, or Acid-Extraction of Meat Products Improves Iron Uptake from Cereal-Meat Product Combinations in an In Vitro Digestion/

Caco-2 Cell Model," *British Journal of Nutrition* 101, no. 6 (2009): 816–821, doi: 10.1017/S000711450805558X.

5 K. M. Redfern et al., "Nutrient-Extraction Blender Preparation Reduces Postprandial Glucose Responses from Fruit Juice Consumption," *Nutrition & Diabetes* 7 (2017): e288.

6 Julie E. Flood and Barbara J. Rolls, "Soup Preloads in a Variety of Forms Reduce Meal Energy Intake," *Appetite* 49, no. 3 (2007): 626–634, doi: 10.1016/j.appet.2007.04.002.

7 Yikyung Park et al., "Dietary Fiber Intake and Mortality in the NIH-AARP Diet and Health Study," *Archives of Internal Medicine* 171, no. 12 (2011): 1061–1068, doi: 10.1001/archinternmed.2011.18.

8 Christina L. Sherry et al., "Sickness Behavior Induced by Endotoxin Can Be Mitigated by the Dietary Soluble Fiber, Pectin, through Up-Regulation of IL-4 and Th2 Polarization," *Brain, Behavior, and Immunity* 24, no. 4 (2010): 631–640, doi: 10.1016/j.bbi.2010.01.015.

9 Nancy C. Howarth, Edward Saltzman, and Susan B. Roberts, "Dietary Fiber and Weight Regulation," *Nutrition Reviews* 59, no. 5 (2001): 129–139, doi: 10.1111/j.1753-4887.2001.tb07001.x.

10 Kristen G. Hairston et al., "Lifestyle Factors and 5-Year Abdominal Fat Accumulation in a Minority Cohort: The IRAS Family Study," *Obesity* 20, no. 2 (2011): 421–427, doi: 10.1038/oby.2011.171.

11 Christina L. Sherry et al., "Sickness Behavior Induced by Endotoxin Can Be Mitigated by the Dietary Soluble Fiber, Pectin, through Up-Regulation of IL-4 and Th2 Polarization," *Brain, Behavior, and Immunity* 24, no. 4 (2010): 631–640, doi: 10.1016/j.bbi.2010.01.015.

12 Marika Lyly et al., "The Effect of Fibre Amount, Energy Level, and Viscosity of Beverages Containing Oat Fibre Supplement on Perceived Satiety," *Food & Nutrition Research* 54 (2010), doi: 10.3402/fnr.v54i0.2149.

13 Julie E. Flood-Obbagy and Barbara J. Rolls, "The Effect of Fruit in Different Forms on Energy Intake and Satiety at a Meal," *Appetite* 5, no. 2 (2009): 416–422, doi: 10.1016/j.appet.2008.12.001.

14 J. Lindström et al., "High-Fibre, Low-Fat Diet Predicts Long-Term Weight Loss and Decreased Type 2 Diabetes Risk: The Finnish Diabetes Prevention Study," *Diabetologia* 49 (2006): 912–920, doi: 10.1007/s00125 -006-0198-3.

CHAPTER 4

1 Camila Domonoske, "50 Years Ago, Sugar Industry Quietly Paid Scientists to Point Blame at Fat," *NPR*, September 13, 2016, https://www.npr.org/ sections/thetwo-way/2016/09/13/493739074/50-years-ago-sugar-industry -quietly-paid-scientists-to-point-blame-at-fat.

2 Anahad O'Connor, "Coca-Cola Funds Scientists Who Shift Blame for Obesity away from Bad Diets," *New York Times,* August 9, 2015, https:// well.blogs.nytimes.com/2015/08/09/coca-cola-funds-scientists-who-shift -blame-for-obesity-away-from-bad-diets.

3 Candice Choi, "How Candy Makers Shape Nutrition Science," *AP News,* June 2, 2016, https://apnews.com/f9483d554430445fa6566bb0aaa293d1/ap -exclusive-how-candy-makers-shape-nutrition-science.

4 Alice Walton, "How Much Sugar Are Americans Eating? [Infographic]," *Forbes,* http://www.forbes.com/sites/alicegwalton/2012/08/30/how-much -sugar-are-americans-eating-infographic, accessed January 29, 2014.

5 Stephen Guyenet and Jeremy Landen, "By 2606, the U.S. Diet Will Be 100 Percent Sugar," *Whole Health Source,* February 18, 2012, https:// wholehealthsource.blogspot.com/2012/02/by-2606-us-diet-will-be-100 -percent.html.

6 World Population Review, "Healthiest Countries 2020," February 17, 2020, https://worldpopulationreview.com/countries/healthiest-countries.

7 B. M. Popkin and C. Hawkes, "Sweetening of the Global Diet, Particularly Beverages: Patterns, Trends, and Policy Responses," *Lancet Diabetes & Endocrinology* 4, no. 2 (2015): 174–186.

8 Marie-Pierre St-Onge et al., "Fiber and Saturated Fat Are Associated with

Sleep Arousals and Slow Wave Sleep," *Journal of Clinical Sleep Medicine* 12, no. 1 (2016), 19–24, doi: 10.5664/jcsm.5384.

9 Linda Rath, "Cancer and Sugar: Is There a Link?," *WebMD*, reviewed February 12, 2019, https://www.webmd.com/cancer/features/cancer-sugar-link#1.

CHAPTER 6

1 Michael Zemel, "The Role of Dairy Foods in Weight Management," *Journal of the American College of Nutrition* 24, suppl. no. 6 (2005): 537S–546S.

2 Carlos Cantó et al., "The NAD(+) Precursor Nicotinamide Riboside Enhances Oxidative Metabolism and Protects against High-Fat Diet-Induced Obesity," *Cell Metabolism* 15, no. 6 (2012): 838–847, doi: 10.1016/j.cmet.2012.04.022; A. R. Josse et al., "Increased Consumption of Dairy Foods and Protein During Diet- and Exercise-Induced Weight Loss Promotes Fat Mass Loss and Lean Mass Gain in Overweight and Obese Premenopausal Women," *Journal of Nutrition* 141, no. 9 (2011): 1626–1634, doi: 10.3945/jn.111.141028.

3 J. Z Ilich et al., "Role of Calcium and Low-Fat Dairy Foods in Weight-Loss Outcomes Revisited: Results from the Randomized Trial of Effects on Bone and Body Composition in Overweight/Obese Postmenopausal Women," *Nutrients* 11, no. 5 (2019): 1157, doi: 10.3390/nu11051157.

4 Heather J. Leidy et al., "Neural Responses to Visual Food Stimuli after a Normal vs. Higher Protein Breakfast in Breakfast-Skipping Teens: A Pilot fMRI Study," *Obesity* (2011): 2019–2025, doi: 10.1038/oby.2011.108.

5 University of Illinois College of Agricultural, Consumer and Environmental Sciences, "Eating Protein throughout the Day Preserves Muscle and Physical Function in Dieting Postmenopausal Women, Study Suggests," *ScienceDaily*, http://www.sciencedaily.com/releases/2011/08/110810153 710.htm, accessed July 25, 2012.

6 D. Paddon-Jones et al., "Protein, Weight Management, and Satiety," *American Journal of Clinical Nutrition* 87, no. 5 (2008): 1558S–1561S.

7 Alison K. Gosby et al., "Testing Protein Leverage in Lean Humans: A Randomised Controlled Experimental Study," *PLoS ONE* 6, no. 10 (2011): e25929, doi: 10.1371/journal.pone.0025929.

8 Jing Zhou et al., "Higher-Protein Diets Improve Indexes of Sleep in Energy-Restricted Overweight and Obese Adults: Results from 2 Randomized Controlled Trials," *American Journal of Clinical Nutrition* 103, no. 3 (2016): 766–774, doi: 10.3945/ajcn.115.124669.

9 American Academy of Neurology, "Alzheimer's: Diet Patterns May Keep Brain from Shrinking," *ScienceDaily*, December 30, 2011.

10 Anwar T. Merchant, et al. "Carbohydrate Intake and Overweight and Obesity Among Healthy Adults." *Journal of the American Dietetic Association* 109, no. 7 (2009): 1165–72, doi:10.1016/j.jada.2009.04.002.

11 N. C. Howarth, E. Saltzman, and S. B. Roberts, "Dietary Fiber and Weight Regulation," *Nutrition Reviews* 59, no. 5 (2001): 129–139.

12 Beth Israel Deaconess Medical Center, "Moderate Coffee Consumption Offers Protection against Heart Failure, Study Suggests," *ScienceDaily*, June 26, 2012.

13 Neil Osterwell, "Health Benefits of Coffee," *WebMD*, August 29, 2011; Youjin Je et al., "A Prospective Cohort Study of Coffee Consumption and Risk of Endometrial Cancer over a 26-Year Follow-Up," *Cancer Epidemiology, Biomarkers & Prevention* (2011): 2487–2495, doi: 10.1158/1055-9965. EPI-11-0766; Fengju Song, Abrar A. Qureshi, and Jiali Han, "Increased Caffeine Intake Is Associated with Reduced Risk of Basal Cell Carcinoma of the Skin," *Cancer Research* 72 (2012): 3282–3289, doi: 10.1158/00085472. CAN-11-3511.

14 Lap Ho et al., "Dietary Supplementation with Decaffeinated Green Coffee Improves Diet-Induced Insulin Resistance and Brain Energy Metabolism in Mice," *Nutritional Neuroscience* 15, no. 1 (2012): 37–45, doi: 10.1179/1476830511Y.0000000027.

15 Liz Szabo, "Coffee Drinkers May Live Longer, Study Suggests," *USA Today*, May 17, 2012.

16 S. L. Schmit et al., "Coffee Consumption and the Risk of Colorectal

Cancer," *Cancer Epidemiology, Biomarkers & Prevention: A Publication of the American Association for Cancer Research* 25, no. 4 (2016): 634–639, doi: 10.1158/1055-9965.EPI-15-0924.

17 G. Pounds et al., "Reduction by Coffee Consumption of Prostate Cancer Risk: Evidence from the Moli-Sani Cohort and Cellular Models," *International Journal of Cancer* 141 (2017): 72–82, doi: 10.1002/ijc.30720.

18 "Drinking Coffee May Be Associated with Reduced Risk of Heart Failure and Stroke," American Heart Association Meeting Report Poster Presentation M2040-Session: LB.APS.o7, November 13, 2017, https://newsroom .heart.org/news/drinking-coffee-may-be-associated-with-reduced-risk-of -heart-failure-and-stroke.

19 J. Li et al., "Habitual Tea Drinking Modulates Brain Efficiency: Evidence from Brain Connectivity Evaluation," *Aging* 11 (2019): 3876–3890, doi: 10.18632/aging.102023.

20 X. Wang et al., "Tea Consumption and the Risk of Atherosclerotic Cardiovascular Disease and All-Cause Mortality: The China-PAR Project," *European Journal of Preventive Cardiology* (2020), doi: 10.1177/2047487319894685.

21 Jenny Hope, "Junk Food Fan? Drinking Tea Could Keep the Pounds at Bay," *The Daily Mail*, December 20, 2010.

22 S. M. Henning et al., "Decaffeinated Green and Black Tea Polyphenols Decrease Weight Gain and Alter Microbiome Populations and Function in Diet-Induced Obese Mice," *European Journal of Nutrition* 57 (2018): 2759–2769, doi: 10.1007/s00394-017-1542-8.

23 E. Weronica et al. on behalf of the Epigenome-Wide Association Study Consortium, "Tea and Coffee Consumption in Relation to DNA Methylation in Four European Cohorts," *Human Molecular Genetics* 26, no. 16 (2017): 3221–3231, doi: 10.1093/hmg/ddx194.

24 F. Haidari et al., "Effect of Green Tea Extract on Body Weight, Serum Glucose, and Lipid Profile in Streptozotocin-Induced Diabetic Rats. A Dose Response Study," *Saudi Medicine Journal* 33, no. 2 (2012): 128–133.

25 Kimberly A. Grove et al., "(–)-Epigallocatechin-3-gallate Inhibits Pancreatic Lipase and Reduces Body Weight Gain in High Fat-Fed

Obese Mice," *Obesity* 20, no. 11 (2011): 2311–2313, doi: 10.1038/oby .2011.139.

26 L. K. Han et al., "Anti-Obesity Action of Oolong Tea," *International Journal of Obesity and Related Metabolic Disorders* 23, no. 1 (1999): 98–105; R. R. He et al., "Beneficial Effects of Oolong Tea Consumption on Diet-Induced Overweight and Obese Subjects," *Chinese Journal of Integrative Medicine* 15, no. 1 (2009): 34–41.

27 H. Shi et al., "Oolong Tea Extract Induces DNA Damage and Cleavage and Inhibits Breast Cancer Cell Growth and Tumorigenesis," *Anticancer Research* 38, no. 11 (2018): 6217–6223, doi: 10.21873/anticanres.12976.

28 Max Roser and Hannah Ritchie, "Food Supply," *Our World in Data*, https://ourworldindata.org/food-supply, accessed April 13, 2020.

29 E. Martínez Steele et al., "Ultra-Processed Foods and Added Sugars in the U.S. Diet: Evidence from a Nationally Representative Cross-Sectional Study," *BMJ Open* 6 (2016): e009892, doi: 10.1136/bmjopen-2015-009892.

CHAPTER 8

1 E. S. Epel et al., "Stress and Body Shape: Stress-Induced Cortisol Secretion Is Consistently Greater among Women with Central Fat," *Psychosomatic Medicine* 62, no. 5 (2000): 623–632.

2 R. S. Paffenbarger et al., "Physical Activity, All-Cause Mortality, and Longevity of College Alumni," *New England Journal of Medicine* 314, no. 10 (1986): 605–613; Gretchen Reynolds, "Moderation as Sweet Spot for Exercise," *New York Times*, June 6, 2012.

3 M. J. Lambiase et al., "Temporal Relationships between Physical Activity and Sleep in Older Women," *Medicine and Science in Sports and Exercise* 45, no. 12 (2013): 2362–2368, doi: 10.1249/MSS.0b013e31829e4cea.

4 Michael J. Wheeler et al., "Distinct Effects of Acute Exercise and Breaks in Sitting on Working Memory and Executive Function in Older Adults: A Three-Arm, Randomised Cross-Over Trial to Evaluate the Effects of Exercise

with and without Breaks in Sitting on Cognition," *British Journal of Sports Medicine* 54, no. 13 (2019): 776–781, doi: 10.1136/bjsports-2018-100168.

5 Michael Thomas, "Exercise Helps Beat the Blues," *Michigan Chronicle,* November 6, 2010.

6 Dennis Thompson, "To Best Fight Cancer, New Guidelines Urge Exercise: Advice Represents Sea Change from 'Take It Easy' to 'Get Moving,'" *Consumer Health News,* November 5, 2010.

7 T. Heir and G. Eide, "Injury Proneness in Infantry Conscripts Undergoing a Physical Training Programme: Smokeless Tobacco Use, Higher Age, and Low Levels of Physical Fitness Are Risk Factors," *Scandinavian Journal of Medicine & Science in Sports* 7, no. 5 (1997): 304–311.

8 C. N. May et al., "Acute Aerobic Exercise Increases Implicit Approach Motivation for Dessert Images," *Journal of Health Psychology* 23, no. 6 (2018): 807–817, doi: 10.1177/1359105316657404.

9 Ing-Mari Dohrn et al., "Replacing Sedentary Time with Physical Activity: A 15-Year Follow-Up of Mortality in a National Cohort," *Clinical Epidemiology* 10 (2018): 179, doi: 10.2147/CLEP.S151613.

10 I. M. Lee et al., "Physical Activity and Coronary Heart Disease in Women: Is 'No Pain, No Gain' Passé?," *Journal of the American Medical Association* 285, no. 11 (2001): 1447–1454.

11 T. Althoff et al., "Large-Scale Physical Activity Data Reveal Worldwide Activity Inequality," *Nature* 547 (2017): 336–339, doi: 10.1038/nature 23018.

12 I. Lee et al., "Association of Step Volume and Intensity with All-Cause Mortality in Older Women," *JAMA Internal Medicine* 179, no. 8 (2019): 1105–1112, doi: 10.1001/jamainternmed.2019.0899.

CHAPTER 9

1 Donna Olmstead, "Give Bones a Boost," *Albuquerque Journal,* August 9, 2009.

2 F. Mayer et al., "The Intensity and Effects of Strength Training in the El-

derly," *Deutsches Ärzteblatt International* 108, no. 21 (2011): 359–364, doi: 10.3238/arztebl.2011.0359.

3 R. A. Winett and R. N. Carpinelli, "Potential Health-Related Benefits of Resistance Training," *Preventative Medicine* 33, no. 5 (2001): 503–513.

4 C. J. Mitchell et al., "Resistance Exercise Load Does Not Determine Training-Mediated Hypertrophic Gains in Young Men," *Journal of Applied Physiology* 113, no. 1 (2012): 71–77, doi: 10.1152/japplphysiol.00307 .2012.

CHAPTER 11

1 M. Murphy et al., "Size of Food Bowl and Scoop Affects Amount of Food Owners Feed Their Dogs," *Journal of Animal Physiology and Animal Nutrition* 96, no. 2 (2012): 237–241, doi: 10.1111/j.1439-0396.2011.01144.x.

2 "Size Can Fool the Eyes: Larger Dishes Can Make It Difficult to Limit Your Portions," *News-Sentinel,* November 25, 2008.

3 Nicholas Bakalar, "Servings: Smaller Scoops May Yield Trimmer Waists," *New York Times,* August 1, 2006.

4 A. McTiernan et al., "Self-Monitoring and Eating-Related Behaviors Are Associated with 12-Month Weight Loss among Postmenopausal Overweight-to-Obese Women in a Dietary Weight Loss Intervention," *Journal of the Academy of Nutrition and Dietetics* 112, no. 9 (2012): 1428–1435.

CHAPTER 13

1 Lora E. Burke, et al. "Self-monitoring in Weight Loss: a Systematic Review of the Literature." *Journal of the American Dietetic Association* 111, no. 1 (2011): 92–102. doi:10.1016/j.jada.2010.10.008.

APPENDIX A

1 M. A. Wien, et al. "Almonds vs Complex Carbohydrates in a Weight Reduction Program." *International Journal of Obesity and Related Metabolic Disorders: Journal of the International Association for the Study of Obesity* 27, no. 11 (2003): 1365–72. doi:10.1038/sj.ijo.0802411.

2 S. E. Berry et al., "Manipulation of Lipid Bioaccessibility of Almond Seeds Influences Postprandial Lipemia in Healthy Human Subjects," *American Journal of Clinical Nutrition* 88, no. 4 (2008): 922–929.

3 Jaapna Dhillon, Sze-Yen Tan, and Richard D. Mattes, "Almond Consumption during Energy Restriction Lowers Truncal Fat and Blood Pressure in Compliant Overweight or Obese Adults," *Journal of Nutrition* 146, no. 12 (2016): 2513–2519, doi: 10.3945/jn.116.238444.

4 Jaapna Dhillon, Sze-Yen Tan, and Richard D. Mattes, "Effects of Almond Consumption on the Post-Lunch Dip and Long-Term Cognitive Function in Energy-Restricted Overweight and Obese Adults," *British Journal of Nutrition* 117, no. 3 (2017): 395–402, doi: 10.1017/S0007114516004463.

5 M. L. Bertoia et al., "Changes in Intake of Fruits and Vegetables and Weight Change in United States Men and Women Followed for Up to 24 Years: Analysis from Three Prospective Cohort Studies," *PLOS Medicine* 13, no. 1 (2016): e1001956, doi: 10.1371/journal.pmed.1001956.

6 Samina Haq and Abir Alamro, "Neuroprotective Effect of Quercetin in Murine Cortical Brain Tissue Cultures," *Clinical Nutrition Experimental* 23 (2018): 89–96, doi: 10.1016/j.yclnex.2018.10.002.

7 C. Puel et al., "Prevention of Bone Loss by Phloridzin, an Apple Polyphenol, in Ovariectomized Rats under Inflammation Conditions," *Calcified Tissue International* 77, no. 5 (2005): 311–318.

8 T. M. Scott et al., "Avocado Consumption Increases Macular Pigment Density in Older Adults: A Randomized, Controlled Trial," *Nutrients* 9, no. 9 (2017): 919, doi: 10.3390/nu9090919.

9 L. Zhu et al., "Using the Avocado to Test the Satiety Effects of a Fat-Fiber Combination in Place of Carbohydrate Energy in a Breakfast Meal in Overweight and Obese Men and Women: A Randomized Clinical Trial," *Nutrients* 11, no . 5 (2019): 952, doi: 10.3390/nu11050952.

10 Nuray Unlu et al., "Carotenoid Absorption from Salad and Salsa by Humans Is Enhanced by the Addition of Avocado or Avocado Oil," *Journal of Nutrition* 135, no. 3 (2005): 431–436.

11 D. J. A. Jenkins et al., "Effect of Legumes as Part of a Low Glycemic Index Diet on Glycemic Control and Cardiovascular Risk Factors in Type 2 Diabetes Mellitus: A Randomized Controlled Trial," *Archives of Internal Medicine* 72, no. 21 (2012): 1653–1660, doi: 10.1001/2013.jamaintern med.70.

12 University of Michigan, "Blueberries May Help Reduce Belly Fat, Diabetes Risk," *ScienceDaily,* April 20, 2009, http://www.sciencedaily.com/releases/2009/04/090419170112.htm.

13 Rosalie Marion Bliss, "Nutrition and Brain Function: Food for the Aging Mind," *Agricultural Research* 55, no. 7 (2007): 8–13.

14 Y. R. Lee et al., "Reactivation of PTEN Tumor Suppressor for Cancer Treatment through Inhibition of a MYC-WWP1 Inhibitory Pathway," *Science* 364, no. 6441 (2019): eaau0159, doi: 10.1126/science.aau0159.

15 A. Ayaz et al., "Chia Seed (*Salvia Hispanica L.*) Added Yogurt Reduces Short-Term Food Intake and Increases Satiety: Randomised Controlled Trial," *Nutrition Research and Practice* 11, no. 5 (2017): 412–418, doi: 10.4162/nrp.2017.11.5.412.

16 Rosalie Marion Bliss, "Researchers Study Effect of Cinnamon Compounds on Brain Cells," USDA Agricultural Research Service, November 9, 2009.

17 Saeideh Momtaz et al., "Cinnamon, a Promising Prospect Towards Alzheimer's Disease," *Pharmacological Research* 130 (2018): 241–258, doi: 10.1016/j.phrs.2017.12.011.

18 A. Bridge et al., "Greek Yogurt and 12 Weeks of Exercise Training on Strength, Muscle Thickness, and Body Composition in Lean, Untrained,

University-Aged Males," *Frontiers in Nutrition* 6 (2019): 55, doi: 10.3389/
fnut.2019.00055.

19 Angela Haupt and Kurtis Hiatt, "Greek Yogurt vs. Regular Yogurt:
Which Is More Healthful?," *U.S. News & World Report,* September 30, 2011.

20 Bamini Gopinath et al., "Dietary Flavonoids and the Prevalence and
15-y Incidence of Age-Related Macular Degeneration," *American Journal of
Clinical Nutritio*n 108, no. 2 (2018): 381–387, doi: 10.1093/ajcn/nqy114.

Index

activity, daily, 97–100. *See also* exercise; resistance training; steps

activity tracker, selecting, 102

alcohol, 79, 161

Almost-Classic 10-Minute Gazpacho, 246–47

Apple Pie Smoothie, 192

apples and pears
  benefits of, 33, 174
  juice vs. blended beverage, 33

Argentinean Steak Salad with Mustard-Cilantro Vinaigrette, 270–71

avocados, benefits of, 174–75

Ball Hamstring Curl, 131

beans, benefits of, 175–76

berries, benefits of, 176

beverages. *See also* smoothies; smoothies and soups, making; soups, blended
  about: coconut water, 76; overview of, 74–75
  alcohol, 79, 161
  coffee/coffee drinks, 76–77
  tea (black/green/herbal/oolong/white), 77–79
  water(s), 75–76

Black Bean and Lime-Mango Salad, 263

Black Bean Soup with Lime, 250–51

blender, 28–29

blender, not having, alternative, 81

blending, 28–37
  bioavailability of food, 30
  juicing vs., 30–32
  liquid meals/energy advantage, 34
  virtues of, 28–30, 32, 34

blood sugar
  alternative sweeteners and, 46–47
  beans stabilizing, 175–76
  cinnamon lowering, 178
  high-fiber carbs and, 71
  smoothies/soups stabilizing, 66
  teas stabilizing, 78

Body Reset Diet. *See also* Phase I; Phase II; Phase III; resistance training *references*; smoothies; smoothies and soups, making; snacks; soups, blended; steps

Body Reset Diet *(cont.)*
    about: new features in this book,
        x–xi; overview of phases,
        53–57; this book and
        changes since first edition,
        vii–xii, 18; why it works,
        17–21
    author's life/qualifications and, x
    benefits, 18–21
    eating habits and, ix–x
    educating you about health/
        fitness, 24–25
    effectiveness of, xi–xii
    exercise and diet trends since
        2013, vii–viii
    expectations, 18–21, 23–25,
        79–80
    health trends and, viii–ix
    length of, 23
    social media and, ix
    solving problems of other diets,
        20–21
    starting, 86
    sugar and, 46, 47–49
    template for, 54
    testimonials, 26–27, 58, 82, 95,
        115, 140, 144, 163, 164–65,
        191
    tips for long-term success,
        163–71
    trusting, 22–23
    uniqueness of, 17–19, 20–21
    weight-loss approach, 19–20,
        170–71
    where to start, xi
    why you can trust, 22–23
Breakfast Burritos I, 228
Breakfast Burritos II, 229
broccoli, benefits of,
    176–77

calories
    chart comparing Phase I to
        average diet, 80
    daily consumption in U.S., 79–80
    excessive restriction, 11, 20
    not created equal, 11, 20
    Phase I totals, 80
cancer, sugar and, 43
carbohydrates, high-fiber, 71,
    91–94. *See also* fiber
Caribbean Kale Smoothie, 206
cauliflower, benefits of, 177
Chicken and Zucchini Salad
    with Buttermilk Dressing,
    266
Chickpea "Tuna" Salad Sandwich,
    234
Chocolate Smoothie, 209
Chopped Greek Salad, 260–61
cinnamon, benefits of, 178
Circuit A, 119–21, 124–32, 141–42,
    154. *See also* resistance
    training
Circuit B, 142–43, 146–54. *See also*
    resistance training
Coconut Chicken Curry, 279
coffee/coffee drinks, 76–77
Cool Cucumber-Lime Smoothie,
    205
crackers (high-fiber), 72
Creamy Black Bean and Pumpkin
    Soup, 252
"Creamy" Cauliflower-Spinach
    Soup, 210
Creamy Spinach and Chickpea
    Stir-Fry, 277
C-snacks. *See* snacks
Curried Cauliflower Soup, 248–49
Curried Turkey and Pear Sandwich,
    240

dairy (milk/yogurt), virtues/
   benefits, 64–65, 178–79
diets
   about: overview of why they fail,
      3–4, 20–21
   apps for fitness and, 6
   Body Reset Diet solutions, 20–21
      (*See also* Body Reset Diet)
   calories and, 11, 20
   confusing basic nutritional
      facts, 11
   costing too much, 8–9, 21
   cutting out entire food category,
      6–7
   exercise balance and, 12–15 (*See
      also* exercise)
   extreme quick fixes, 4–5
   health coaching and, 4
   ignoring pleasure of eating, 10
   intermittent fasting, 9
   ketogenic, x, 6–7
   listening to the wrong people, 4
   meal replacement products and,
      5–6
   scale not dropping fast enough,
      15–16, 20
   taking too much time, 8, 20
   teaching wrong lessons, 10
   weight-loss pills and, 5
   yo-yoing on, 7–8
Dijon Lentil Salad with Baby
   Spinach, 265

Easy Niçoise Salad, 268
eating. *See also* ingredients
   habits, ix–x
   mindfully, 164
   planning meals, 113–14, 138–39,
      163
   portion control, 84, 136–38

restoring passion for, 109–10
schedules (*See* menus and
   schedules)
slowly, 164
tips for long-term success,
   163–71
exercise. *See also* resistance training
   references; steps
   activity tracker and, 102
   daily physical activity
      importance vs., 97–100
   differentiating activity from, 99
   excessive, 12, 96
   extreme trends, vii–viii, 96
   maintenance mode movement
      guidelines, 57
   Phase I movement guidelines,
      55, 101–4, 169
   Phase II movement guidelines,
      56, 116, 132, 169
   Phase III movement guidelines,
      57, 134, 154, 169
   regular movement and, 14
   rest of your life, 169–70
   sedentary lifestyle and, 14–15,
      99–100
   spinning in perspective, 97
   sticking to your plan, 168–69
   too little, diets and, 13–15
   too much, diets and, 12–13, 97, 98
   trendy fitness products and, 15
expectations, for Body Reset Diet,
   18–21, 23–25, 79–80

Fall Fruit Frosty, 196
fasting, intermittent, 9
fat, healthy, 69–71, 91
fiber
   blending vs. juicing and, 30–33
   digestion and elimination, 36

fiber *(cont.)*
   facts and benefits, 34–37
   high-fiber carbs for
      smoothies/soups, 71,
      91–94
   soluble vs. insoluble, 36–37
   weight loss and, 34–35
flavor accents, 94
food prep basics, 110–13
free meals, 21, 46, 49, 57, 160–63,
     166, 167
fruits
   about: blending vs. juicing,
      30–33; fiber factor, 34–37;
      health and nutrition
      benefits, 39; high-fiber
      for smoothies, 91–92; for
      snacks, 72; sugar contents
      (highest and lowest), 92–93;
      virtues of blending, 28–30,
      32, 34

Ginger Shrimp with Chard and Bell
     Peppers, 280–81
Golden Split Pea Soup, 257
grazing vs. gorging, 9, 19–20
Greek Tuna Melt, 243
Green Mango Smoothie, 203
Green Soup, 188–91
Grilled Steak and Baby Spinach
     Salad, 264

hamstring curls, 130–31
Harley's Hearty Egg Muffin, 227
Harley's Potato-Pepper Easy
     Omelet, 222–23
Herbed Cream Cheese Scramble,
     224–25
Homemade Gyros, 244–45
Homestyle Chicken Soup, 256

immunity, sugar and, 42
inflammation, sugar and, 42
ingredients (smoothie/blended
     soup), 62–71. *See also*
     smoothies and soups,
     making
   about: the case for milk/yogurt,
      64–65; cleaning house,
      165–66; flavor accents,
      94; for perfect smoothies,
      63; shopping list, 84–88;
      stocking up, 165
   alphabetical listing with their
      benefits, 173–82
   category #1: liquid base,
      66–67, 90
   category #2: lean protein, 67–69,
      90–91
   category #3: healthy fat,
      69–71, 91
   category #4: high-fiber carbs, 71,
      91–94
ingredients, other. *See* beverages;
     snacks
insulin sensitivity, sugar and, 42
intermittent fasting, 9
Italian Flag Breakfast Pizza, 220–21

juicing, blending vs., 30–32

ketogenic diets, x, 6–7
Kiwi-Strawberry Smoothie, 204
Kung Pao-ish Chicken, 274–75

leafy greens, for smoothies/blended
     soups, 93
Lemon Quinoa with Spring
     Vegetables, 267
Lemon Ricotta Edamame Crostini,
     238

limes, benefits of, 179–80
liquid base, for smoothies/soups,
     66–67, 90
Lying Triceps Extension, 127

maintenance mode, 157–71
   about: diet and movement
        overview, 57; overview of,
        157–58
   free meals, 21, 46, 49, 57, 160–63,
        166, 167
   hitting reset again, 159
   tips for long-term success,
        163–71
Maxwell Mocha Smoothie, 207
meal prep, 110–13
meal replacement products
        (MRPs), 5–6, 81
mental health, sugar and, 43
menus and schedules
   about: keeping things simple,
        167–68; setting schedule,
        88–89; sticking to schedule,
        166–67
   menu overview Phases I, II,
        III, 56
   Phase I movement schedule,
        169
   Phase I sample menu, 104
   Phase II movement schedule,
        132, 169
   Phase II planning and menu
        guide, 113–14
   Phase III movement schedule,
        154, 169
   Phase III planning and menu
        guide, 138–39
   plan for rest of your life, 167
Mexican Chicken Salad with Spicy
        Salsa Dressing, 269

milk
   as liquid base, 66–67, 90
   nondairy, 67, 90
   virtues/benefits, 64–65
Modified Push-Up, 148–49
movement. See exercise
muscles, strengthening. See
        resistance training; steps

9-Minute Shrimp and Asparagus
        Stir-Fry, 272–73
nutrition
   bad vs. good fats, 70
   blending vs. juicing and, 30–33
   diets confusing facts about, 11
   expectations for this diet, 24
   healthy fat and, 69–71
   for smoothies/soups, 89 (See also
        specific recipes)
nuts and seeds
   almond benefits, 173–74
   chia seeds benefits, 177–78
   as healthy fat ingredients, 91

Onion, Turkey Sausage, and
        Spinach Frittata, 218–19
Open-Faced Chicken and
        Caramelized Onion
        Sandwich, 242
Open-Faced Egg and Bacon
        Sandwiches, 232
oranges, benefits of, 180

passion for eating, restoring,
        109–10
PB&J Smoothie, 200
Pear Spice Smoothie, 195
Phase I. See also smoothies;
        smoothies and soups, making;
        snacks; soups, blended

Phase I *(cont.)*
  about: overview of, 55; what
        you'll be doing, 61; what
        you'll need, 62
  calorie expectations, 79–80
  daily movement guidelines, 55,
        101–4 (*See also* exercise)
  diet overview, 55, 56
  movement/steps guidelines, 55,
        101, 103, 169
  sample schedule, 104
  shopping list, 84–88
  starting, 86
  sugar and, 47–48
Phase II, 107–32. *See also* resistance
        training *references*
  about: overview and summary,
        55–56, 107–9, 132; what
        you'll be doing, 107, 132;
        what you'll need, 108
  biggest dietary change, 108
  diet overview, 55–56
  food prep basics, 110–13
  going to 12,000 steps, 116, 132
  menu guide, 114
  movement/steps guidelines, 56,
        116, 132, 169
  planning meals, 113–14
  restoring passion for eating,
        109–10
  transitioning back to single-dish
        meals, 108, 109–10, 114–15
Phase III, 135–54
  about: overview and summary,
        56, 135–36, 154; what you'll
        be doing, 135, 154; what
        you'll need, 136
  diet overview, 56
  life after (*See* maintenance
        mode)

menu guide, 139
movement/steps guidelines,
        56, 135, 154, 169 (*See
        also* resistance training
        references)
planning meals, 138–39
portion control, 136–38
pills, weight-loss, 5
Piña Colada Smoothie, 208
Plank, 152–53
planning meals
  long-term success and, 163
  Phase II, 113–14
  Phase III, 138–39
popcorn, 73
portion sizes, controlling, 84,
        136–38
prepping meals, 110–13
Prone Hamstring Curl, 130
protein (lean)
  animal sources, 67
  functions and need for, 68–69
  powder, benefits and selecting,
        180–81
  for smoothies/blended soups,
        67–69, 90–91
  vegetarian sources, 67–68, 90–91
push-up, modified, 148–49

Quesadilla Master Recipe, 235–36

Raspberry–Lemon Drop Smoothie,
        201
recipes. *See also* ingredients; S-
        meals *references* (salads,
        sandwiches, scrambles,
        soups, stir-fries); smoothies;
        smoothies and soups,
        making; snacks (C-snacks);
        soups, blended

ease and simplicity of, 110–13
food prep basics, 110–13
getting creative, 158–59
other books for, 112
S-meals explained, 112–13
Red Smoothie, 186–87
reset, 15-day. *See* Phase I; Phase II;
    Phase III; resistance
    training *references;*
    smoothies; smoothies
    and soups, making;
    snacks; soups, blended;
    steps
reset, hitting again, 159
resistance training, 116–32
    alternating Circuit A and
        Circuit B, 142, 143
    anterior muscles, 142 (*See also*
        Circuit B)
    Circuit A, 119–21, 124–32,
        141–42, 154
    Circuit B, 142–43, 146–54
    correcting muscle imbalances,
        142
    exercises (*See* resistance training
        exercises *references*)
    fitness levels, 120
    frequency of, 121, 143
    increasing the resistance,
        141–44, 146–54
    intensity levels, 117–18
    no equipment needed, 118
    Phase II, 119–21, 132, 169
    Phase III, 141–43, 169
    posterior muscles, 119 (*See also*
        Circuit A)
    purpose and benefits, 117, 121,
        141–42
    repetitions and number of
        circuits, 120–21, 143

schedule, 132
time required for, 118, 141
resistance training exercises
    (Circuit A), 124–31
    #1: Reverse Fly, 124–25
    #2: Triceps Dip or Lying Triceps
        Extension, 126–27
    #3: Superman, 128–29
    #4: Prone Hamstring Curl or Ball
        Hamstring Curl, 130–31
resistance training exercises
    (Circuit B)
    #1: Squat or Skater Lunge,
        146–47
    #2: Modified Push-Up, 148–49
    #3: Standing Side Bend, 150–51
    #4: Plank, 152–53
rest of your life. *See* maintenance
    mode
Reverse Fly, 124–25
rhabdomyolysis, 13
Roast Beef and Caramelized Onion
    Wrap, 237
Ruby Red Frosty, 197

salads. *See* S-meals (salads)
sandwiches. *See* S-meals
    (sandwiches)
schedule. *See* menus and schedules
scrambles. *See* S-meals (scrambles)
Sesame Red and Green Slaw, 262
Shaved Sprouts Salad, 258–59
shopping list, 84–88. *See also*
    smoothies and soups,
    making
Shrimp and Noodle Stir-Fry, 282
Shrimp and Rice Stir-Fry, 284
side bend, standing, 150–51
single-dish meals, transitioning back
    to, 108, 109–10, 114–15

Skater Lunge, 147
Skinny Mint Pea Soup, 211
sleep, sugar and, 42–43
S-meals
    definition and types of meals,
        112–13
    transitioning back to, 108,
        109–10, 114–15
S-meals (salads), 258–71
    Argentinean Steak Salad
        with Mustard-Cilantro
        Vinaigrette, 270–71
    Black Bean and Lime-Mango
        Salad, 263
    Chicken and Zucchini Salad
        with Buttermilk Dressing,
        266
    Chopped Greek Salad, 260–61
    Dijon Lentil Salad with Baby
        Spinach, 265
    Easy Niçoise Salad, 268
    Grilled Steak and Baby Spinach
        Salad, 264
    Lemon Quinoa with Spring
        Vegetables, 267
    Mexican Chicken Salad with
        Spicy Salsa Dressing, 269
    Sesame Red and Green Slaw,
        262
    Shaved Sprouts Salad, 258–59
S-meals (sandwiches), 233–45
    about: overview of, 233
    Chickpea "Tuna" Salad
        Sandwich, 234
    Curried Turkey and Pear
        Sandwich, 240
    Greek Tuna Melt, 243
    Homemade Gyros, 244–45
    Lemon Ricotta Edamame
        Crostini, 238

    Open-Faced Chicken and
        Caramelized Onion
        Sandwich, 242
    Open-Faced Egg and Bacon
        Sandwiches, 232
    Quesadilla Master Recipe,
        235–36
    Roast Beef and Caramelized
        Onion Wrap, 237
    Southwestern Tuna Tortilla
        Wrap, 239
    Tzatziki Chicken Flatbread, 241
S-meals (scrambles), 218–32
    Breakfast Burritos I, 228
    Breakfast Burritos II, 229
    Harley's Hearty Egg Muffin,
        227
    Harley's Potato-Pepper Easy
        Omelet, 222–23
    Herbed Cream Cheese Scramble,
        224–25
    Italian Flag Breakfast Pizza,
        220–21
    Onion, Turkey Sausage, and
        Spinach Frittata, 218–19
    Open-Faced Egg and Bacon
        Sandwiches, 232
    Sweet Potato Home Fries and
        Eggs, 226, 230–31
S-meals (soups), 246–57
    Almost-Classic 10-Minute
        Gazpacho, 246–47
    Black Bean Soup with Lime,
        250–51
    Creamy Black Bean and
        Pumpkin Soup, 252
    Curried Cauliflower Soup,
        248–49
    Golden Split Pea Soup, 257
    Homestyle Chicken Soup, 256

Sunset Squash Soup, 253
Winter's Day Beef with Barley
    Soup, 254–55
S-meals (stir-fries), 272–84
    Coconut Chicken Curry, 279
    Creamy Spinach and Chickpea
        Stir-Fry, 277
    Ginger Shrimp with Chard and
        Bell Peppers, 280–81
    Kung Pao-ish Chicken, 274–75
    9-Minute Shrimp and Asparagus
        Stir-Fry, 272–73
    Shrimp and Noodle Stir-Fry, 282
    Shrimp and Rice Stir-Fry, 284
    Spicy Beef Stir-Fry, 283
    10-Minute Stir-Fry, 276
    Tuscan White Bean and Kale
        Bruschetta, 278
smoothies, 183–211. *See also*
    ingredients (smoothie/
    blended soup); smoothies
    and soups, making
    about: adaptability of recipes, 89;
        the case for milk/yogurt,
        64–65; MRP options in
        lieu of, 81; red smoothies,
        197–201; stabilizing blood
        sugar, 66; sugar and, 62;
        white smoothies, 192–96
    Apple Pie Smoothie, 192
    Caribbean Kale Smoothie, 206
    Chocolate Smoothie, 209
    Cool Cucumber-Lime Smoothie,
        205
    "Creamy" Cauliflower-Spinach
        Soup, 210
    Fall Fruit Frosty, 196
    Green Mango Smoothie, 203
    Kiwi-Strawberry Smoothie, 204
    Maxwell Mocha Smoothie, 207

PB&J Smoothie, 200
Pear Spice Smoothie, 195
Piña Colada Smoothie, 208
Raspberry–Lemon Drop
    Smoothie, 201
Red Smoothie, 186–87
Ruby Red Frosty, 197
Stonefruit Smoothie, 199
Sweet Spinach Smoothie, 202
Tropical Morning Smoothie, 194
Very Berry Smoothie, 198
White Peach Ginger Smoothie,
    193
White Smoothie, 184–85
smoothies and soups, making. *See
    also* ingredients (smoothie/
    blended soup)
    about: adaptability of recipes,
        83–84; assembling
        and benefits, 62–66;
        components for perfection,
        63; diet and movement
        overview, 84; nutrition/
        calorie objectives, 89; white
        and red smoothies, green
        soups, 83
    getting creative, 158–59
    portion control and, 84
    step 1: make shopping list, 84–88
    step 2: set a schedule, 88–89
    step 3: build the smoothies/
        soups, 89–94
snacks (C-snacks)
    about: guidelines, 72–73, 88, 213;
        shopping list, 88
    crackers (high-fiber), 72, 214,
        215
    eating with protein, 73
    examples (complete and combo),
        73–74, 213–15

snacks (C-snacks) *(cont.)*
  fruits, 72
  popcorn, 73
social media, ix
soups, blended. *See also* ingredients
      (smoothie/blended soup);
      smoothies and soups,
      making
  about: assembling and benefits,
      62–66; daily routine by
      phase, 56; shopping list, 86;
      stabilizing blood sugar, 66;
      vegetables and, 62–66
  Green Soup, 188–91
  Skinny Mint Pea Soup, 211
soups, other. *See* S-meals (soups)
Southwestern Tuna Tortilla Wrap,
      239
Spicy Beef Stir-Fry, 283
spinach, benefits of, 181–82
Squat or Skater Lunge, 146–47
Standing Side Bend, 150–51
starting diet, 86
steps
  activity tracker for, 55, 102
  getting 10,000 steps, 101–3
  going to 12,000 steps, 116,
      132
  minimum daily/magic number,
      55, 56, 101–3
  Phase I, 55, 101–3, 169
  Phase II, 56, 116, 132, 169
  Phase III, 56, 135, 154, 169
  year-round/rest of your life, 57,
      169–70
stir-fry meals. *See* S-meals
      (stir-fries)
Stonefruit Smoothie, 199
success tips, long-term, 163–71
sugar, 38–49

alternative sweeteners and,
      46–47
Body Reset Diet and, 46, 47–49
brain and, 41–42
cancer and, 43
consumption statistics, 39–40
in fruit, highest and lowest levels,
      92–93
hidden sources and names of, 41,
      44, 45
ill effects on body, 40–43
immunity and, 42
inflammation and, 42
insulin sensitivity and, 42
kinds of, 44
as main health culprit, 38–39
mental health and, 43
reducing, 44, 46–47
sleep and, 42–43
smoothies and, 62
weight gain/loss and, 39, 43
Sunset Squash Soup, 253
Superman, 128–29
Sweet Potato Home Fries and Eggs,
      226, 230–31
Sweet Spinach Smoothie, 202
sweeteners, alternative, 46–47, 48
Sweetkick, 48

tea, 77–79
template, reset, 54
10-Minute Stir-Fry, 276
testimonials, 26–27, 58, 82, 95, 115,
      140, 144, 163, 164–65, 191
Triceps Dip or Lying Triceps
      Extension, 126–27
Tropical Morning Smoothie, 194
Tuscan White Bean and Kale
      Bruschetta, 278
Tzatziki Chicken Flatbread, 241

vegetables
  about: best for smoothies and
        soups, 93–94; blended
        soups and, 62–66; blending
        vs. juicing, 30–32; fiber
        factor, 34–37; flavor
        accents, 94; leafy greens, 93;
        virtues of blending, 28–30,
        32, 34
Very Berry Smoothie, 198

water(s), 75–76
weight loss
  Body Reset Diet approach,
        19–20, 170–71
  denying yourself of food
        and, 19

diets and rate of, 15–16
expectations for this diet,
        23–25
grazing vs. gorging, 9,
        19–20
liquid energy and, 34 (*See also*
        blending)
long-term view, 39
sugar and, 39, 43
White Peach Ginger Smoothie,
        193
White Smoothie, 184–85
Winter's Day Beef with Barley
        Soup, 254–55

yogurt, virtues/benefits, 64, 65,
        178–79

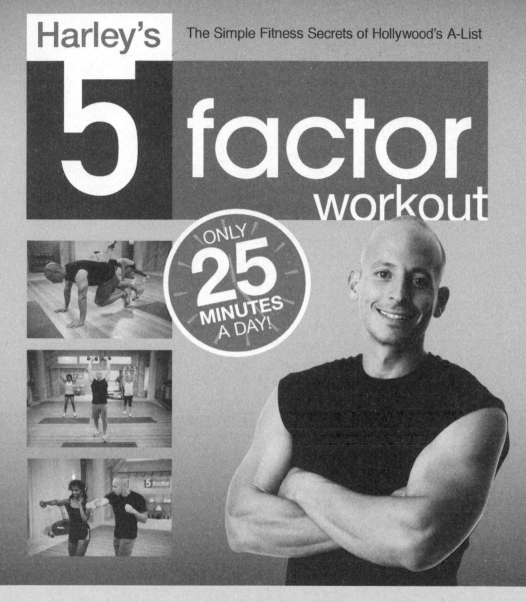

Harley's

5 factor workout

The Simple Fitness Secrets of Hollywood's A-List

ONLY **25** MINUTES A DAY!

From Hollywood to your home, get direct access to the world's top celebrity trainer, whose 25-minute-a-day workout will give you a celebrity body in just five weeks!

Now Available on DVD and Digital Download
More info at www.newvideo.com/harley

NEWVIDEO
A CINEDIGM COMPANY